PRAISE FOR *Th*

"Tracee Stanley has gifted the world with another incredible and one-or-a-kind resource that is filled with countless gems of her grounded and embodied wisdom. *The Luminous Self* is an experiential and restorative guidebook that reminds us that Yoga is truly a state of being and that our spiritual practices and rituals are a sacred way of reconnecting us to our deepest selves. With compassion, nuance, and profound magic (in the way only Tracee can do), this book introduces us to the life-shifting practices of ritual, embodiment, movement, meditation, rest, and Yoga nidra. Deeply nourishing and simultaneously awakening—you will not be the same person when you are finished."—ZAHABIYAH YAMASAKI, author of *Trauma-Informed Yoga for Survivors of Sexual Assault*

"Tracee Stanley is emerging as a global leader in the realm of a new and needed embodied spirituality. *The Luminous Self* allows us to penetrate life's deepest and most transcendent question—*Who am I?* She adeptly walks us into the murky ground of this inquiry through both new and time-tested yogic technologies that allow us to release our old identities while simultaneously honoring our body, ancestry, and past experience."—KATIE SILCOX, author of *Happy, Healthy, Sexy*

"Tracee Stanley's teaching is pure transmission; the clarity of her self-respect is of benefit to us all. *Luminous Self* carries us to the heart with applicable, profound practices, providing a structure to nourish both intimacy and freedom within ourselves."—ELENA BROWER, author of *Practice You*

"There are practices and teachings within this book that will change the course of your destiny. *The Luminous Self* is a portal to the inner realms where anything is possible"—KIM KRANS, artist and creator of *The Wild Unknown Tarot*

"It is time to collectively wake up and remember who we are before our forget-fulness causes any more harm to us, all sentient beings, and the planet. *The Luminous Self* is not only a book—it is already a good Ancestor who whispers to us, 'This, this is the way.' You are not lost; follow the ray that points toward the luminous Self."—OCTAVIA RAHEEM, author of *Pause, Rest, Be*

"This work of art speaks to the undoing that meets us all at our proverbial front door when we dive into an inquiry and practice how to heal ourselves and find peace amid a chaotic world and landscape. Tracee provides a soft container that feels like the wisest guidance for the unraveling and undo-ing as well as practices and tools for the journey back into wholeness and truth."—MICHELLE C. JOHNSON, author of *We Heal Together*

"*The Luminous Self* is a bright and effulgent light in the darkness. With com-passion and courage, Tracee Stanley carves away our confusion regarding these ancient, esoteric spiritual teachings to reveal what has been there all along: We are already whole and full. The light we're seeking is within us."—JIVANA HEYMAN, author of *Yoga Revolution*

"Tracee Stanley's book arrives in an age when people are thirsting for an au-thentic path to the true Self. This beautiful and deep book is the dip of cool water needed to slake that thirst."—ACHARYA SHUNYA, author of *Sovereign Self*

The Luminous Self

SACRED YOGIC PRACTICES AND RITUALS
TO REMEMBER WHO YOU ARE

Tracee Stanley

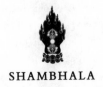

SHAMBHALA

Shambhala Publications, Inc.
2129 13th Street
Boulder, Colorado 80302
www.shambhala.com

Cover art: iStock.com/mycola
Cover & interior design: Kate E. White

9 8 7 6 5 4 3 2 1

First Edition
Printed in the United States of America

Shambhala Publications makes every effort to print on acid-free, recycled paper.
Shambhala Publications is distributed worldwide by Penguin Random
House, Inc., and its subsidiaries.

LIBRARY OF CONGRESS CATALOGING-IN-PUBLICATION DATA
Names: Stanley, Tracee, author.
Title: The luminous self: sacred yogic practices and rituals to
remember who you are / Tracee Stanley.
Description: First edition. | Boulder, Colorado: Shambhala, [2023] |
Includes bibliographical references.
Identifiers: LCCN 2022055370 | ISBN 9781645471660 (trade paperback)
Subjects: LCSH: Yoga. | Self. | Mind and body. | Meditation.
Classification: LCC RA781.67 .S725 2023 | DDC 613.7/046—dc23/eng/20230106
LC record available at https://lccn.loc.gov/2022055370

Om jyotir aham
I am the light of pure consciousness

Contents

Conclusion: Initiate Yourself—Rituals of Power   151

Introduction

THE ETERNAL QUESTION

Early in my life as a spiritual student, over two decades ago, I was sitting in front of a teacher in a private session. We talked about how my yoga practice was going, the obstacles in my life, and the troubles in the relationship I was in at the time. As I was speaking, the teacher took a deep breath and let out a sigh that caused me to pause. He closed his eyes; a silence came over the room as he was motionless for several minutes. I was uncomfortably perched on my chair, a bit dubious, waiting for his next words and wondering what he was doing. When he finally opened his eyes, he looked at me with deep concern and a tinge of sadness and said, "I am not sure that you have ever tasted your true nature."

Immediately several questions popped into my mind: *What does that even mean? How the heck would you know? What is true nature? How will I know when I taste it? What am I? Who am I? WHO AM I?*

This was an inquiry seeking a deeper understanding of Self, a transitional moment in my spiritual journey. Until then, I had been practicing yoga asana to get physically stronger and nail handstands and calming my mind with meditation. I was performing yoga poses but ignorant to the fact that there is no "doing" yoga. Yoga is a state of being. This question dropped me right into the space of something unknown. A question I had never asked myself. My mind could not think its way to the answer. The power of one question—*Who am I?*—dropped into my awareness in a moment of stillness, and presence was the ripple that shifted the course of my life. In that moment, I became a seeker.

The beauty of my questioning is that it was self-imposed. The teacher's question to himself, wrapped in a statement to me, initiated me into a self-inquiry that I didn't know I needed. The desire to know my true Self was ignited. It is a desire that I believe, deep down, we all share. As I went down many paths to try to find my true Self, I began to realize that no one could answer this for me. Each time I glimpsed a tiny shard of inner light or truth, it seemed more like an unveiling of something ancient that was revealed to me in moments of surrender, deep inquiry, or profound joy and awe. There was an ebb and a flow of revealing and concealing until I learned to slow down and be more present.

This path to the true Self was one of remembrance, and there were (and continue to be) many beliefs, stories, and fears in the way of my remembering and reclaiming my true Self. Along the way, some practices began to crack the shell and pieces of light began to shine through. It is with humility that, in these pages, I share a bit of my journey and the practices that continue to lead me to a deeper exploration of Self.

Let's take a moment to explore the term *true Self*. This is Self with a capital *S*, referring to our inner essence, the part of us that is eternal and unchanging. This true Self is beyond name and form, or what is referred to in Sanskrit as *namarupa*. Namarupa is what makes up our *living* being. *Nama* is the mental aspect, and *rupa* is the physical form, but we are more than just mind and matter. There is a part of us that is beyond gender; it was there before you had a name and will be there when you no longer have a body; it is beyond all conditioning and all sorrow and is more effulgent than the brilliance of the sun, moon, stars, and planets; it permeates the states of consciousness—

waking, dreaming, and deep sleep. This place within us is said to reside in the lotus of our heart and is referred to in Yoga Sutra 1:36. True Self is referred to by many names: Atman, Purusha, soul, inner self, deeper self, inner knowing, inner truth, eternal truth, and inner wisdom. You may notice these descriptions are used interchangeably throughout the book. Remember, when we refer to the true Self, we are speaking about our unchanging eternal essence, not our identity as a human person, which may include race, gender, sexual preference, and so forth. Spiritual teachings should not be used to deny or oppress the radiant expression of any person's inner light in this human form.

Below are two beautiful translations of Yoga Sutra 1:36. I suggest exploring other translations to find the ones that resonate most with you, as it is important for us to remember that truth, light, and wisdom lie within us.

Yoga Sutra 1:36: viśokā vā jyotiṣmatī.[1]
Concentration may also be attained by fixing the mind upon the Inner Light, which is beyond sorrow.
—*Translated by Swami Prabhavananda and Christopher Isherwood*[2]

Or the mind can also find peace by contemplating the luminous light, arising from the heart which is the source of true serenity.
—*Translation by Mukunda Stiles*[3]

NO, THAT'S NOT ME

I am forever grateful for that meeting in a cramped, dusty little office in a seemingly inauspicious building because, at the time, I thought I knew who I was. I had a solid sense of self (notice the lowercase *s*). But if I wasn't the Black female Hollywood film producer, yoga student, homeowner, partner, dog mom, vegetarian, Bermudian American, Francophile, amateur photographer, lover of the ocean, avid reader, and former punk rock kid, who was

I? I had memories of how these identities supported how I showed up in the world—my front-facing little self was on point. I spent countless hours reinforcing these parts of myself that I wanted the world to see. But there was also great pain, shame, grief, and fear tucked below the surface. My inner light was concealed by a veil of forgetting. I made myself just busy enough to forget the pain and suffering was there. And I forgot—at least I thought I did. The problem is there is no actual forgetting. The true Self always remembers; it knows both the cause and the cure. This deepest part of our being holds the wisdom from lifetimes and is constantly sending us the messages to wake up and remember that we are so much more than we think we are.

That teacher was right: I had not tasted my true Self. So the question lingered: Who am I when I leave my successful Hollywood job, get divorced, close my yoga studios, and almost go bankrupt? All these outer identities were masking something; they pointed to the external "I," not the true inner Self. I would come to find out that my attachment to who I wanted the world to see was causing me pain yet also held the power to reveal a great truth.

It is difficult to reclaim the space needed to reflect on the deeper Self when there is a continuous flow of information that leads us to believe that everything we need to be happy is found outside of us. We can be made to feel irrelevant unless we have the latest phone, an impressive résumé, or a youthful appearance. Others may shower us with respect and love if we have the exclusive material possessions and accomplishments that the dominant culture has decided are worthy. To make money, advertisers and marketers use the fact that we are disconnected from our true Self. Motivational research, a psychological marketing technique developed in the 1950s, is a series of protocols designed to uncover consumers' unconscious behaviors, beliefs, and motives that will lead them to purchase a product. We are constantly being marketed to, and that incessant stream of advertising and information is targeted to our unconscious minds. Corporations know more about our core desires and beliefs than we do! Our emotions, fears, and desire to belong are influential factors motivating us to act.

What if we knew who we were at our core essence? What if the outer I authentically reflected our inner Self? How would our lives change? How would our relationships shift? What work would we choose to do or not do? What could we reclaim about ourselves that we thought was lost long ago? What would we remember about our place in the world and the underlying unity of all life?

When we lack the knowledge of our true Self, we lean into trying on the character traits of who others think we should be and what social norms say is "right." We stop dancing to the song of our own soul. We might look outside of ourselves for clues to define who we are or get swept up in what everyone else seems to be doing—just look at the "trends" on TikTok. We can lean into the kind of materialism, ideology, and tribalism that reinforce an outer sense of I-am-ness and keeping us distracted, separate, causing us to continue neglecting our inner Self. Forgetting our true Self can also lead to the intolerance of others who are shining and unapologetic in their expression of their inner light and joy. When we know our true Self, we have compassion, understanding, and contentment; when we don't, we can fall into jealousy, comparison, and even hatred. That sense of I-am-ness in yogic teachings is known as *asmita*, and it is considered one of "the five afflictions" (*kleshas*) that cause us pain and suffering.

REMEMBER WHO YOU ARE

The practices in this book are shared to amplify sacred remembrance of the deeper Self, supporting a transformation from living with the virus of self-forgetting and collective amnesia to awakening to our luminous Self. Self-remembrance is a sacred practice, a prayer, a deep longing, and a journey of self-initiation. Mythologies of many cultures have stories of those who embark on journeys to seek treasures only to realize that what they were seeking was inside them all along. We must remember the power within us.

The need to remember who we are may seem odd, but the true Self is waiting to be recognized. Peeling back the layers that cover our inherent beauty and power might be the most important journey of our lives. If we are brave enough to follow the call inward, we can find a sense of freedom from the obstacles in life that keep us bound in suffering and conflict. We also will find clues that can help us to see the source of our desire to keep others in suffering because we ourselves are disconnected from our inner knowing and power.

This path of sacred remembrance is not about seeking your life's purpose but awakening a deep inner knowing that the north star you have been looking for has been inside you all along. This inward journey is a self-initiation into a sustained connection to your deepest Self. Opportunities, relationships, creative projects, and magic will magnetize toward you when you act in ways that are aligned with who you KNOW yourself to be.

THE PATH

Over the last twenty-seven years, I have done many sadhanas. Those practices consisted of mantras, *kriyas* (yogic technique), and rituals for spiritual awakening, protection, abundance, purification, and healing. The practices and studying I have done in the lineages of the Himalayan tradition and Sri Vidya Tantra have informed my life and teaching in immeasurable ways, and I am grateful for having received their grace. Study in those lineages awakened my curiosity to explore other traditions that also center a connection to the earth, an innate divine force within us, and the interconnectedness of all life. You will notice threads of other wisdom traditions that I have found to be supportive weaving throughout this book. These practices served as tenderizers for my heart to open from the deep contraction I didn't know was there and receive greater wisdom about the nature of my true Self. When I began to share these practices as a teacher, I witnessed powerful shifts and transformations within those who devoted time to practicing them.

This book is an offering of my understanding and experience of the philosophies and practices that I have found most supportive, awakening, and nourishing in my teaching and personal practice. My intention is to share these things in ways that help the modern householder. If you have the responsibility of supporting yourself, caregiving, or raising a family, these practices can help you to sustain a spiritual practice that enriches life.

These practices are meant to be accessible, welcoming, and affirming. Take what works for you and leave the rest. I didn't write this book as a quick fix or a hack to enlightenment. In my experience, spiritual practice blossoms with devotion, consistency, inquiry, and curiosity. I offer these practices as a way to explore, weave, pray, and expand, so that we may shake off the dust of being asleep to our power and ignite awareness of our inherent luminosity. This can be slow medicine, and a new awareness can powerfully descend in an instant. The journey toward remembrance is not linear—offer yourself grace.

HOW TO USE THIS BOOK

In part one, we will begin by taking a deep dive into obstacles to Self-remembrance, exploring power, personality, forgiveness, memory, and understanding of the elements of nature within you as ways to dissolve potential roadblocks. For our most authentic Self to be revealed, it is helpful to acknowledge the old stories, pain, and beliefs that the little self likes to hold on to. This section includes yogic philosophy, self-inquiry, visualization, and community care practices to help us root out the seeds of suffering and awaken to the inherent wisdom within us. You will want to have a journal or notebook to accompany you on this journey. Often in practice we will have a breakthrough or insight; writing it down will help to keep the experience fresh. The ritual of writing (or drawing) after practice helps us to integrate the wisdom we receive by revitalizing our power of retention.

Each chapter in part two is a portal to a deeper awakening. I have included practices and contemplations, sourced from various traditions, that may help you to peel back layers of stagnation to reveal more of your inner essence. My suggestion is to first do the practices in the order they are presented so that they can spark a cumulative momentum. Take your time with all that is offered here—let it marinate. Revisit them more than once over time and see what shifts.

Practices: Each chapter is supported by practices that connect to the theme it explores. The offerings are a tapestry of ritual, movement, meditation, rest practices, yoga nidra, purification practices, and contemplation. Each practice offers suggestions on how it can be modified and adapted for accessibility. Find what works for you and your body. You will also find additional practices at the back of the book to help support your journey.

See, Sense, or Trust: We all have different ways of experiencing life through our five senses. We are often guided in meditation practices to imagine or visualize things in meditation—for example, light or celestial objects. You will notice an instruction to "see, feel, or trust" during the practices in this book. We are not all able to visualize, and there is nothing wrong with your practice if you don't "see" things. Notice what works best for you: see (visualize, imagine), sense (feel, notice, perceive), or trust (have faith even though you may not see or feel anything in the moment). Faith is one of the most essential parts of practice.

Self-Inquiry: Self-inquiry is the way to remember who we are at our essence—the inner I or true Self. The questions provided are meant to support you in finding out. At the deeper level of self-inquiry, we may be asked to trace our thoughts back to their origin beyond the concept of "I" that weaves through every thought and deludes us into believing the ego and personality is who we are.

The great sage Sri Ramana Maharshi became enlightened at sixteen when he had a sudden fear of death. Instead of letting the fear envelop him, he began to watch the process and ask *what* was going to die. Who is the one that is going to die? What will remain? Through this process, he was led to the inner I—the true Self.[4]

The provided questions are contemplations that can create a fertile ground for us to expand awareness by cultivating *smriti* (memory) and follow the thread of inquiry and thought back to its source. Whenever we practice self-inquiry, we should remember Sri Ramana Maharshi.

Rituals: We create rituals in every moment, whether we are conscious of them or not. The rituals we create through unconscious habits become spells that we cast over our lives. The way we think about ourselves, our worth and our potential, cause us to expand or contract in life. Our lives will transform if we become more intentional and present with the habits, thoughts, and actions that we repeat consistently. The late African teacher and writer Sobonfu Somé said, "The purpose of rituals is to take us to a place of self-discovery and mastery. In this sense, ritual is to the soul what food is to the physical body."[5] Rituals will help you to honor, remember, reclaim, and tend to the forgotten parts of yourself. The rituals offered here will support you in the liminality of the transition we experience during any transformational journey. Ritual is the fascia that holds the center when it seems like everything else is falling apart. A daily ritual is a cumulative practice that buoys and nourishes us on every level and is a powerful way to continue to weave the thread of practice through our lives. Ritual is our link to the unseen forces of healing.

Community Care: Our healing is connected. The journey of our healing and remembrance is not just for us. It holds the potential for collective healing if we are intentional and compassionate in our practices. When we offer the benefits of our practice to the sacred collective, our practice extends beyond our limited personal universe and expands far and wide. The author Prem Prakash reminds us in their translation of the Bhakti Sutra that practice limited to a desire for individual accomplishment reinforces "the egoistic knot of separative consciousness that spiritual practice is intended to untie."[6] Suggestions for how to be a force of healing in your family and community are offered as ways to bring an authentic sense of connection, love, and beauty into the web of life.

Support: The support of your sangha, therapists, trusted friends, and family can be invaluable resources during a period of transformation and self-examination. I highly recommend seeking the support of those you trust if difficult or unexpected emotions arise as you move through this book.

Audio Recordings: Six audio practices are available online to guide you. Visit www.shambhala.com/TheLuminousSelfPractices to access them. I recommend listening to the practices first and letting my voice guide you. As you become more familiar with them, you'll be able to guide yourself.

FOR TEACHERS

When I wrote *Radiant Rest: Yoga Nidra for Deep Relaxation and Awakened Clarity*, I wanted it to be an open resource for everyone to cultivate a relationship with yoga nidra, as the feminine power of rest and a state of consciousness that is "peace beyond words."[7] The teachings I share here have touched and transformed me and thousands of those who have practiced with me. This book you hold in your hands now is also an open resource to be shared. The practices I offer have either been shared with me or have come through me. Either way, I am the creator of nothing. I am a vessel to share the wisdom that has touched me. Please receive and share these practices as sacred. *The Luminous Self* isn't a system or protocol but offerings to be embodied and lived. Teachers, please remember powerful transmission comes from embodied wisdom, which means knowing when, how, and where to share and with whom. My suggestion for teachers is to live with and learn from each of these practices for sixty to ninety days each before sharing them. Embrace an attitude of partnering with these practices to experience the wisdom they offer as opposed to trying to extract a result that can be quickly duplicated in a classroom setting. If you do, you will learn things that can never be expressed in words, but the experiences will live through you. Take time to explore the resource material and notes. Sitting with your mentor, teacher, or therapist is also a great idea to process the effects of the practices. Thank you for joining me here. Thank you for your curiosity and courage.

May we remember the sages who first realized the
  light of the true Self.
May we offer gratitude to all teachers, ancestors, and guides
  who continue to light our path toward awakening.
May we know the universe within our hearts.
May we nourished by a deep well of love.
May we all be free.

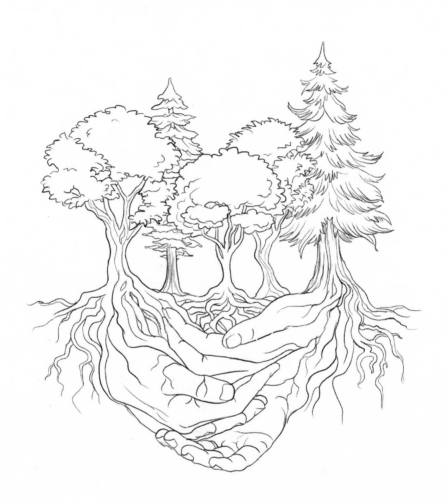

Reclaiming Your Power

The experience of being

A letting go of doing

A presence

Eyes seeing beyond the forms

Ears hearing the vibration of light

Every sense pulsing in and out

A dance

Of knowing and forgetting

Of trusting and doubting

Of grasping and releasing

Now just let me remember when I have forgotten

Beauty is transparent

I see truth in divine connection

Knowing is already here

I am whole and connected

I am supported within and without

Let everyday be a remembrance

a reclaiming

of truth

—Tracee Stanley

TRANSFORMATION IS A JOURNEY toward wholeness and freedom. What transforms one heart has the power to transform many hearts. Part one of this book is a journey toward remembering our wholeness and softening the edges of who we think we are. I present the offerings in a cumulative way that can help peel back layers of stuckness, doubt, and forgetfulness, allowing some light to shine through. Every healing journey is like a unique and personal labyrinth. The path may be narrow, requiring you to be aware of every step. There will be moments of pause and reflection, joy, frustration, inspiration, and resistance, knowing you have not yet arrived at the center. As you move through this book, notice if there is a sense of inner urgency to complete all of the practices and read quickly. That is a signal to slow down and notice what is truly arising. The fast pace of life has trained some of us to want instant gratification, lack patience, and ignore our deepest truths. It's important to honor your process. If a practice doesn't feel right for you at any time, trust your wisdom, freewrite about how you are feeling, and then skip it. Transformation and Self-remembrance require the spaciousness to integrate, expand, reveal, double back, and heal. It is not uncommon to experience resistance when doing practices that can help you to reclaim and trust your inner power. We have spent many years being sold narratives that tell us that worthiness is something to be achieved. Yet denying our inherent worthiness is a self-abandonment that leads to the feeling of someone knocking on a door from our insides, asking us to wake up and open the door to free them. The true Self is always knocking—can we hear them? It is possible that feelings of excitement and resistance may coexist as you move through the practices; let everything you experience be the fuel that sparks the inner alchemy to transform you. If difficult or challenging emotions arise, take time for a longer pause and sit with a trusted mentor or therapist to help you navigate your healing process. Remember to always offer yourself grace.

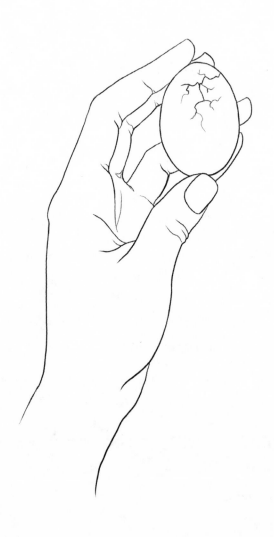

| 1 |

THAT WHICH MAKES YOU FALL IS
THAT WHICH MAKES YOU RISE

HOW DID I FIND MYSELF in my bathroom naked, covered in egg yolk, banging on a drum, screaming and shouting at the top of my lungs? I had just cracked a raw egg over my head. And I had never felt so powerful and fierce. As I stared at myself in the mirror, I saw clarity and resolve in my eyes. I felt free. I knew I had released a power in me that was ancient.

Years of doing spiritual practices led me to this point of self-initiation that marked the moment I resolved to take back my power. It was a ritual, a reclaiming of a part of me that I had forgotten. The power of my deepest Self was waiting to be revealed, renewed, and nurtured.

The face looking back at me in the mirror wasn't much different from that of the eleven-year-old who had stood in the junior high school bathroom in Huntington, New York, several decades earlier covered in broken eggshells, streaks of bright-yellow yolk dried against my dark brown skin. Three girls had just attacked me on the school bus. They didn't like the way I wore my hair, the way I spoke, or the way I dressed. They didn't like anything about me. And they had been diligent in making sure that I knew it every day of the school year. From the first day I put on my first pair of thick eyeglasses in the third grade, I had been bullied. I became used to the name-calling—"Olive Oyl," "Four-Eyes," "Ugly," "Stick Figure"—but there was something different about these girls. They wanted to physically hurt me.

The day before what I'll refer to as the "egg incident," one of the girls watched me walk onto the school bus, turned toward me, and said loudly enough for everyone to hear, "Why do you wear your hair like that? It's ugly!" She was mocking my natural hair that was awkwardly styled in an afro that had been locked in curlers the night before.

As I gathered my things to get off at my bus stop, there was a lot of whispering and snickering. I had a foreboding feeling in the pit in my stomach that something terrible was about to happen; they were planning to do something to me, and I heard a voice say, "Watch out for them."

The next day I thought about trying to get out of going to school, but I knew I would only be putting off the inevitable. So I got myself ready. As I walked the half block to the bus stop, I felt like I was watching myself in a movie, getting ready to walk the plank. Every step was in slow motion and terrifying as I imagined what they might be planning. I wondered if this would be the "sticks and stones" that I had long feared.

As the bus arrived, the creaky doors opened like the mouth of a shark waiting to swallow me. I climbed the steps and noticed that the three girls who usually sat at the back of the bus were up front that day. They all smiled strangely at me, as if to say, *It's alright, don't worry.* But my nervous system knew better, and my heart began to race. I braced myself as I noticed the only open place to sit—one seat behind them. The whole bus seemed to be in on whatever was about to happen. Even my friends wouldn't make eye contact. Then it happened. They jumped me, attacking me—one from behind and the other two from the top, smashing raw eggs into my hair as they cackled and called me names.

No one on the bus did anything, not even the driver. I saw the driver look back, but he just kept going. I tried to protect myself from their blows to the head and face, hoping to keep my glasses from being broken. When

I finally managed to kick the biggest girl off me, I hit her in the head. She looked surprised and then returned to her seat. It was over. I was covered in raw eggs, and they seemed satisfied with the job they had done.

When we arrived at school, I made my way to the nearest bathroom. There I was, one of the youngest seventh graders in the school, standing in the bathroom feeling humiliated and shamed. I had never experienced this kind of public embarrassment before. I still had to make it to my homeroom class. In my imagination, everyone in the entire school had now heard what had happened and was waiting to laugh at me in the big, circular lobby where they hung out before homeroom.

I needed a plan. At the time, my mother was studying Egyptology, and I had been reading her books on the subject. I decided that I would pretend I was Cleopatra, dressed in her finest jewels and robes. I cleaned as much of the egg off as I could; I walked out of the bathroom and down the hall toward my class. I held my head high, shoulders back and chest lifted, as if I was walking through my kingdom. I was Cleopatra. I kept my gaze forward, not looking at anyone. I could feel the stares and snickers, but I ignored them and managed to make it to my class.

During homeroom, I was called to the principal's office. To my surprise, the bus driver had reported the incident, and the principal wanted to know which girls had jumped me. I wouldn't tell. I needed to keep my mouth shut and not risk another attack for telling on them.

The egg incident changed me. I started sitting in the back of the class. I stopped wearing my glasses, even though I couldn't see the board to take notes. I started turning in my homework late or not doing it at all. I was dropped from Honors English and was barely passing French—my two favorite subjects. I gave up playing the clarinet and violin. I stopped being the little girl who loved to learn and excel in school. I was shrinking. And most disturbingly, I started obsessively pulling out my hair, an anxiety condition known as trichotillomania that was misdiagnosed as an infection of hair follicles. The misdiagnosis allowed me to hide my hair pulling for years.

The events of that day were traumatic and had a ripple effect throughout my life that I didn't understand until I began to practice and study the teachings of yoga. Yoga began to slow me down enough to understand that my life decades later was very much being informed by the pain of the past. The egg incident created what is known in yogic teachings as a samskara, an impression or imprint.[1] *Everything* we experience in life creates an imprint; in the journey of remembering our true nature, this is a concept we should explore and understand. We will take a deep dive into these concepts and how they shape our lives in the next chapter.

INTENTIONAL PAUSE: CONNECT TO YOUR BREATH

Take a moment of intentional pause. If it's comfortable, close your eyes or soften your gaze. Place your hands on your belly. Welcome three deep belly breaths—in through your nose, out through your mouth with an audible sigh. Then receive

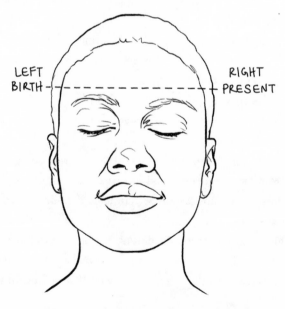

three deep breaths in through your nose and out through your nose. Feel your belly rise and fall as you breathe in and out.

Maybe in your life you've had a moment like mine—a demarcation moment, when something shifted within you because of an impactful emotional experience. It could be a moment of great joy and pride or a moment of deep sadness, fear, or discomfort. Life is a ceaseless flow of impressions and sometimes they can be challenging to navigate. If you have experienced trauma, it may be helpful to discuss your insights and feelings with a trusted therapist as you explore the next practice.

SELF-REFLECTION PRACTICE: TIMELINE REWIND—TRACING THE IMPRESSIONS
(10 minutes)

We will begin this practice by exploring the remembrance of peacefulness as an impression. Practice this contemplation sitting up in your preferred meditation shape.

Close your eyes if that is available to you; if not, keep your eyes slightly open and lower your gaze to the floor. Begin by gently bringing awareness to your breath. Notice your breath as it enters your nostrils; be aware of the cool temperature of your breath. As your breath leaves your nostrils, notice your breath is warmer. Repeat for three breaths, aware of the flow and temperature of your breath with each inhale and exhale.

Feel your belly expanding as you inhale and contracting as you exhale. Allow your chest to become still. Sense that all of your breath moves into your belly as the chest becomes still. For ten breaths, continue to feel your navel rise and fall. Allow your breath to be effortless, smooth, and even—that is, inhalation and the exhalation of equal length. This is 1:1 ratio breathing. For example, inhale for four counts and exhale for four counts. Feel into the space your body occupies from the top of your head to the tips of your toes. Feel as though your whole body is breathing. (1 minute)

Be aware of the space around your body. Draw a circle of protective light around your body. Choose any light that feels most protective to you—for example, fire or moonlight. If it is helpful, you can request benevolent beings or guides to surround the circumference of this circle to bring an additional layer of protection and peace to your circle of energetic protection. (1 minute)

Bring your awareness back into the space inside your body and feel into the space inside your head. Imagine the inside of your head as empty space—no organ or bones, just empty blank space.[2]

Bring your attention to your right ear and feel as though you can draw a line from your right ear all the way to your left ear through the empty space of your head.

Feel and sense this line as a timeline of your life. Your right ear represents this present moment, and your left ear represents the moment you were born. As you feel into this timeline, begin at the right ear, pausing to recall the most recent experience where you felt a sense of peace. Just let your mind quickly rest in that moment in time; see or sense a snapshot of where you were and what you were doing in this peaceful moment. Don't get caught up in a story—just remember the moment. And then quickly move on from the right ear toward the left ear as you move backward on the timeline to the next profound moment of peace, again just experiencing a snapshot of this moment in time and continuing to move backward, touching all of the significant moments

Continue to move backward in time toward your left ear until you reach another significant moment. Go back as far as you can in time until you reach the first moment you felt profound peace. If at any time you begin to feel uncomfortable, pause the practice and ground yourself by going outside for a walk or lying on the ground for a few minutes doing deep belly breathing.

When you feel complete, please spend five minutes freewriting about what you remembered and how you feel. In freewriting, you write whatever comes to mind as quickly as you can, without attention to sentence structure or spelling. Do not disregard any memory as insignificant. If the memory entered your awareness, it's meaningful.

When your writing feels complete, take a moment to notice if there was any recurring theme among the memories that popped up for you. Write it down.

As you traced your life back to reexperience moments that created impactful impressions of peace, you may have encountered a variety of emotions. You may find this exercise helpful to trace back other impressions like courage, joy, discomfort, fear, or inspiration. The first time I did this practice I traced back the impressions of shame throughout my life, and it was helpful for me to understand how samskaras have shaped me. It's important to acknowledge the impact of tracing the impressions on our timeline. The emotions that arise may be surprising, and you may need a moment to reset; please take a moment to transition from the last exercise by shaking it out.

INTENTIONAL PAUSE:
JIBBA JABBA—SHAKING IT OUT
(10 minutes)

Shaking is a practice that helps to regulate the nervous system. You may notice that your dog shakes to release tension or stress.[3] It is important for us to give ourselves space to release emotions, anxiety, and stuck energy. When we shake, we mimic the body's innate response to discharge overwhelm in the nervous system.[4] When we add sound to accompany our movement, we give voice and physical expression to thoughts and feelings that can otherwise be difficult to name and release.

Set your timer for five minutes.

Find a comfortable position standing. You can also do this practice lying down or sitting in a chair if standing or walking is not accessible for you. Begin by slowing walking in a small circle, moving your arms as you move.

Next, begin to repeat "Jibba jabba!! Jibba jabba!!" over and over to represent all the thoughts, worries, and concerns of the mind. By using "jibba jabba," we let go of the idea of connecting to a story and can begin allowing thoughts and emotions to be released and spaciousness to be created. As you continue, get louder and louder with your jibba jabbas, beginning to shake your whole body as much as is available to you—especially the arms, hands, feet, and legs. Shake every part of your body that is possible to shake. If you can't shake any part of the body, *imagine* the body shaking. Continue walking (or jogging) faster in your circle and shaking it out while repeating "Jibba jabba!! Jibba jabba!!"

After three minutes of shaking and jibba jabbas, pause and be silent.

Lie down. Rest and notice your body lying on the floor. (2 minutes)

Let your breath settle back into your belly. Watch the rise and fall of your navel. (1 minute)

Devote a few minutes to freewriting.

"That which makes you fall is that which makes you rise": I first heard this wisdom from the tantric teacher Sally Kempton, and it immediately reminded me of a verse from Coleman Barks's translation of the poem "Childhood Friends" by the thirteenth-century Persian poet Jalal al-Din Rumi:

Don't turn your head. Keep looking at the bandaged place. That's where the light enters you.[5]

What if we examined our wounded places with compassion and acceptance? Could we see how we were shaped by them? Our reaction to painful experiences is nuanced, and we should be careful not to judge ourselves or measure our experience against another person. We can be both strengthened by these experiences and feel stuck in place at the same time.

There were a few things that were set in motion the day of the egg incident. The feeling of "watching myself in a movie" as I walked onto the school bus was the first experience that I can recall of witness consciousness—the feeling of being a detached observer of my thoughts and feelings. I learned that I had a powerful intuition, even though it would take me years to learn to trust it.

One of the gifts of that day was that I learned how to be resilient, but I also became less trusting. I began to study martial arts, and by eighteen I had a purple mohawk and spent Sunday afternoons stagediving at CBGB. I was physically strong, and my outer appearance said, *You better not mess with me.* But was that the real me? Or was I just wearing a mask?

INTENTIONAL PAUSE: SELF-INQUIRY

Devote several minutes to answering the following inquiries:

- What gifts or seminal lessons have you received from challenging experiences in life? Do these lessons have an expansive or contracting expression?
- What past experiences and wounds are you ready to heal from?
- Can you trace a limiting belief that you currently hold to an impactful experience of the past? This is where the Timeline Rewind Practice might be helpful (see page 9).

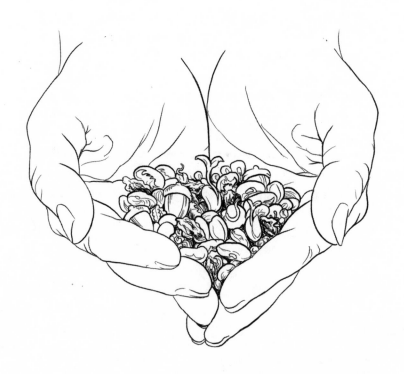

| 2 |

YOU ARE NOT YOUR PERSONALITY

THE ETYMOLOGY OF THE WORD *personality* comes from the Latin *persona*, which refers to a theatrical mask used by actors to disguise their true identities.[1] Think of all the masks that YOU have put on over the years. Which ones have you forgotten to take off? Does your mask feel like a warm invitation or a rhino's armoring? Exploring the makeup of our personality is an essential part of remembering the power and radiance of who we are at our core essence. My egg incident was an experience that gave rise to new habits and ways of being that I used to protect myself against future pain. They concretized over time to shape a personality that was much different from who I was before. That version of me went unchallenged for decades until I asked the essential question—Who am I? Once I began to investigate my personality, I was able to see how seeds of experience that were planted long ago had propelled me to act in certain ways and to form beliefs about the world and my place in it that limited my potential. A worldview informed by pain and shame held me back from remembering my full self. Our personality consists of a cluster of our habits, which are formed by life experiences and our memory of them. This cluster is a coloring that obscures the true Self.

The teachings of yoga give us ways to understand how experiences can and do shape our lives. The sage Patanjali, who is said to have been born sometime between the second and fourth centuries C.E., codified the oral teachings of the ancient rishis (original seers of yoga) into 196 aphorisms. The Sanskrit word *sutra*, which has the same Latin root as *suture*, refers to a thread that is woven through a text to connect and build on wisdom that reveals truth. Patanjali's Yoga Sutras have four chapters that illuminate paths that lead to spiritual freedom respectively. Patanjali introduces the concepts of how our personalities are formed in the first chapter of the Yoga Sutras, the Samadhi Pada, which is dedicated to enlightenment, ways to clear the mind, and obstacles to yoga. It is important to note that the study of Patanjali's Yoga Sutras would take many lifetimes. What I offer in these pages is a way to explore and introduce the concepts. You will find resources to deepen your study of the Yoga Sutras on page 185. Let's take an imaginary trip together to dive deeper into these concepts.

THE ROAD TRIP OF LIFE

Imagine the moment you are born. You arrive full of potential. Whether born prematurely, in poverty, in illness, or in radiant health, there is a part of you that is eternal and infinitely luminous, untouched by external conditions. There is an eternal place within each of us that is said to be effulgent and beyond all sorrow.[2] This luminosity is not earned or granted to us in some merit-based system. It is inherently part of us and more brilliant than the sun, moon, and all the light in the galaxies, but it is veiled from our awareness. Remembering the luminous part of ourselves is part of our spiritual journey and a purpose in life.

At the beginning of the road trip, you are behind the wheel of your vehicle and marvel at the big panoramic windshield in front of you. You get started on the long road trip of life. You are full of infinite potential, and your vehicle has a special GPS configured to help you navigate life's roads. That GPS is constantly sending you signals and signs of how to stay on course to return to remembering your true Self. That internal GPS is the wisdom of your soul, otherwise known as your intuition.

If you have ever been on a long road trip, you know about the inevitable first bug splat on the windshield. Remember that everything we experience in life creates an impression, or samskara. Those impressions are like splats on the windshield, and they happen all the time. Scraping your knee at age five creates an impression. Learning to ride your bike creates an impression. Your grandmother dying creates an impression. Learning how to safely cross the street creates an impression. Falling in love creates an impression. Being betrayed creates an impression. Being told you're a failure creates an impression. Experiencing the unconditional love of a pet creates an impression. In my egg incident, being attacked for thriving as my uniquely nerdy self created an impression. Our life is a sequence of countless impressions and imprints. There is no way to escape them, so we file them away, categorizing them as good, bad, or neutral. Our windshield is constantly covered. What is on our windshield? How is it affecting our life? How can we gain clarity and reconnect to our innate gifts and wisdom?

You may remember some of the memories that showed up on your screen of awareness during the Timeline Rewind practice in the previous chapter. Each of those memories is formed from a samskara, the bug colliding with your windshield. Some of the bugs make little splats, and others make the kind of huge yellow gooey splatters that make you think to yourself, *I definitely have to wash my windshield at the next gas station!* But then at the gas station there is a distraction—some chocolates you really want, an email dinging, your child needing your attention—and you forget to wash the windshield. Off you go then, continuing your journey with a dirty windshield. You try the next gas station, and there are no resources or tools to wash your windshield—no water, no squeegee, no attendant to give you a hand. So you keep driving, and it just keeps accumulating more and more bugs. You try the windshield wipers and it creates a giant smear. Now you can't really see what is in front of you. All you see is a coloring. What you see through the windshield does not accurately represent what is out in front of you. You have lost clarity, perception, and vision. You can barely see the road ahead. After a long while, you forget that the windshield was ever clear. That dirty windshield seems perfectly normal. You have forgotten that you have an internal GPS because it is obscured by the coloring, and your attention is focused externally.

You keep driving and reacting according to what you see on the windshield instead of the reality of what's ahead of you. At this point you may not even be on the road any longer. You become a prisoner to the coloring that is now on the windshield. That coloring is known as *vasana*, an accumulation of imprints that form a coloring of the mind. This coloring gives rise to habits or actions based on your response to the coloring. If the coloring stays on for too long, the habits become concretized and become our personality. We then become attached to our personality because we have forgotten who we really are. We have forgotten our radiance. We believe that our personality is the whole of who we are and forget that we are wearing a mask, made up of all the coloring of life's experiences. This can lead to suffering. In yogic philosophy, the cause of suffering is known as *avidya*, or misperception, ignorance, wrong knowledge. Your dirty windshield has caused you to make wrong turns and decisions because you are in ignorance of your true nature, and you lack clear sight.

This dirty windshield and the habits you have formed by looking through it have now informed and concretized into your personality and your worldview, affecting how you see the world, what you believe about it, and how you react to it. You may find yourself experiencing the same things over and over and seemingly never learning the lesson. You never stop to ask yourself, *What lesson am I tired of learning and why do I keep having the same undesirable outcomes in life?* An unseen force is compelling you to continue driving, though you have forgotten why you are driving or even where you might be headed. Every once in a while, you may have a moment when you think you hear a voice or you get inspired to make a turn in a new direction. Still, something might hold you back from following through to the magical destination of infinite possibilities that is just over the pass.

It's easy to forget that there is something great waiting for us when all we see is a dirty windshield. We need tools to get back on track, practices to remind us that we are not the car, the bugs, or the windshield. We are radiant, infinite potential, and our true Self is waiting for us to remember. The moment we realize that we have lost our way, or have lost clarity, is a moment of transition. We have sparked a desire to find ourselves again. We know that something must change. We need to remember who we really are and begin to act accordingly. But how?

No one can do the kind of windshield cleaning you need for you. A great psychotherapist can guide you (see resources in the back of the book), but ultimately you must do the work. You have to be the one to scrub the sticky caked-on coloring off of the windshield so you can see again. Don't worry—you don't have to do it all at once. All you need is one tiny spot to begin to gain some clarity and momentum.

POWER-WASHING THE WINDSHIELD

Self-reflection, meditation, and deep relaxation practices are like a power wash for our windshield. We cannot escape impressions and the colorings created, as they are always happening. But we can begin to burn the seeds of samskara, making them less potent or inert. And we can reduce the coloring on the windshield. You'll need a handful of tools to begin cleaning your windshield spot by spot.

INTENTIONAL PAUSE: SELF-INQUIRY

Devote a few minutes for the following questions:

- How are your accumulated samskaras leading to discomfort or stuckness in your life?
- Do you feel as though you are at a transitional point in your life? What

ways of being are you ready to release? How would you like to see your
life change?

WHO AM I NOT?

Imposter syndrome is a psychological term referring to a pattern of behavior
where people doubt their accomplishments and have a persistent, often internalized fear of being exposed as a fraud. Not an actual disorder, the term
was coined by the clinical psychologists Pauline Clance and Suzanne Imes in
1978, when they found that despite having adequate external evidence of accomplishments, people with imposter syndrome remained convinced that they
don't deserve the success they have.

—*Psychology Today*[3]

Most people who describe experiencing imposter syndrome share that they
feel like they are "faking it," they don't "know" enough, they need one more
training or certification to prove that they can do the thing. It's a pervasive
feeling in our society, and it directly relates to our exploration of personality. Let's reframe that last sentence of the description of imposter syndrome
quoted from *Psychology Today*—despite having adequate evidence that we
possess intuition, unique genius, and wisdom, people with imposter syndrome deny the call of the true Self, ignoring their insights, creative muses,
and inner knowing; they are convinced that they don't deserve to experience the inherent joy and power that accompanies sharing their distinct gifts
with the world.

The world has us believing that we are so unworthy and incapable of
fulfilling our dreams and passions that we ignore of the whispers of our soul.
When we step out of the automatic pilot zone of being asleep to our genius
and into the space of intuition and deep listening, we can become petrified
because the inner spaciousness that emerges feels so foreign to us. The source
of resistance will remain clouded unless we acknowledge that there is resis-

tance and then ask ourselves, Who is the real imposter? Is it the you who tries to conform and compete with what everyone else is doing, the you who feels the urgency to stay relevant within the ever-changing trends that the world dictates as worthy and desirable? Or is it the you who has had a flash of inspiration and insight and wants to follow that flow of energy and share your unique light with the world? Which part of you feels like the imposter—the personality that is formed of your habits, vasanas, and samskaras or the part of you that desires know wholeness and freedom? How are you abandoning your Self to fit in?

INTENTIONAL PAUSE: SELF-INQUIRY

Consider the following questions:

- What part of you feels like a fraud or an imposter?
- When do you feel most at ease and authentic? When do feel safe to share your authentic self? When do you feel the need to hide?
- How do you neglect your unique gifts in the world? What dream do you have for yourself that you have never shared with anyone?

Your inner luminosity is calling you to awaken to your full power and clarity. The dullness of collective amnesia propels us toward mediocrity and lack of fulfillment. Despite us wanting to live our "best life," we can feel stuck, and the biggest resistance to us following through on the call of our heart is doubt. Doubt is a form of resistance to remembering our true Self and our inherent power; it shows up in many forms—distraction, fear, procrastination, and the outsourcing of our knowing and creativity to others. It is easy to doubt the wisdom of the true Self when we are emmeshed in the prison of the lower mind. The practices of self-inquiry and contemplation are some of the tools that can begin to loosen the grip of samskaras. Remember the essential question: Who am I? In yogic practice, it is important to explore the opposite of things, whether they be emotions, thoughts, or ideas. The following practice asks you to explore the two sides of the coin.

WHO AM I NOT? PRACTICE
(30 minutes)

You will need a mirror, voice recorder, and notebook. Set a timer for five minutes, start your voice recorder, and stand in front of the mirror.

Part 1: Seeing (7 minutes)

Place one hand on your belly and the other hand on your chest. Practice centering 1:1 diaphragmatic breathing. (2 minutes)

Open your eyes and begin to gaze into your own eyes in the mirror; do not break the gaze with yourself until the exercise is over.

Ask yourself the following questions, answering quickly:

- Who am I?
- Who am I not?
- Who am I?
- Who am I not?

Continue this for five minutes, asking and answering as quickly as you can. It doesn't matter if the answers make sense. Don't think about; just keep going.

When the timer goes off, move on to part 2 of the practice.

Part 2: Remembering (2 minutes)

Create a two-column list in your notebook. Label the first column "Who Am I?" Label the second column "Who Am I Not?" Begin to recall from memory your answers and write them in the corresponding columns.

Who Am I?	Who Am I Not?

Part 3: Listening (5 minutes)

Listen back to the recording of yourself doing the exercise. Add any answers that you missed to your lists.

Part 4: Accepting (3 minutes)

Now review your list and make notes. Which of these answers feel like labels or personality traits? Which answers feel the most like your core essence, essential truth, or expression of your authentic Self? There are no wrong or right answers. This practice is a peeling back, a revealing, and you can come back to it many times, or practice it as a daily sadhana for nine consecutive days.

Part 5: Learning (3 minutes)

What did I see? What did I hear? What did I learn? Devote a few moments to freewrite reflections on these questions as they relate to the exercise and any insights you may have received.

- What did you see in your eyes as you gazed at yourself in the mirror? Did you find it challenging to hold presence with yourself?

- What did you hear in your voice?
- What did you learn from this practice?

Part 6: Rest (10 minutes)

Allow yourself to rest, take a nap, or practice deep relaxation for a few minutes after you finish this practice. Resting will allow you to deeply integrate the practice. When your rest is complete, dedicate a few additional minutes to freewriting.

INTENTIONAL PAUSE: SELF-INQUIRY

Take a moment to consider:

- What labels, jobs, or responsibilities are you ready to release?

PURIFYING OUR NEGATIVE TENDENCIES

As we explore our personality, we get to see what is on our windshield and discern what is helpful for us and what isn't. This is where the practices of laya yoga come to our aid. *Laya* means "dissolution" and refers to a body of practices that help us to dissolve the grossest form of something so that we can reduce it to a subtler form and realize its origins. Laya yoga is alchemy for the soul, as it slowly reveals the hidden, golden self deep within us. Laya yoga practices work on the level of the subtle body—the interconnected layers of energy that make up our being beyond the physical form. Tantric teachings tell us there is a universe that exists inside of each of us. Science has affirmed what the rishis knew long ago—that everything in the universe is also found in our bodies; we are made of stardust.[4] Beginning to explore our personal inner cosmos and the subtle energies within us will have a transformative effect on our outer life. Tantric philosophy tells us that all of creation is comprised of *tattvas*, or "thatness." The understanding of the tattvas allows us to understand the nature of reality. Our awareness of own true nature then naturally expands as we are a reflection of all creation. We can begin this understanding by working with the five tattvas, or elements—earth, water, fire, air, and space/ether.

TRANSFORMING PERSONALITY PRACTICE

The purification and dissolution of the elements within ourselves ignites transformation and expansion of consciousness. The following practice is a simplified version of a laya yoga practice that I learned many years ago that asks you explore the embodiment of negativity within you. The practice can be very revealing in just one sitting. However, I suggest practicing this, along with freewriting, consistently over a forty-day period, as the efficacy of the practice is cumulative, like many practices in tantra. Done over a long period of time, it can support you in your understanding of what it means to move awareness from gross to subtle.

The first step of this visualization is to consider a negative aspect of your personality that you would like to transform. That's a big question. Likely the answer may have already popped into your mind. Pause and notice if you have resistance to answering this question. If you are having trouble deciding, ask yourself, *What part of my personality has consistently caused me the most discomfort?* Take a moment to consider the personality trait that you would like to work with before continuing. You'll find some examples below.

Jealous

Unforgiving

Judgmental

Dishonest

Manipulative

Having a lack of boundaries

Selfish

Not speaking up for myself

Domineering

Fearful

INTENTIONAL PAUSE:
A PRAYER FOR HEALING AND WISDOM

Take a moment to take three deep breaths and offer gratitude for the sages and the five elements. Take a moment to visualize or connect with each of the elements—earth, water, fire, air, ether. Take another moment to say a prayer for your healing: "I offer myself grace. May I find healing and wisdom in this practice."

MINDFUL MOVEMENT

3–5 minutes

Please spend several minutes moving your body with gentle, conscious movement, asana, or dancing. Listen to your body. Connect your breath with your movement, bringing presence and intention into your body. You can find suggestions for movement practices on page 162.

As you begin this meditation, have your journal nearby. Find a comfortable meditative seat with your spine relatively perpendicular to the earth. If that is not available to you, it is fine to support yourself in a chair, against a wall, or propped up in your bed.

Note: Doing this practice in a completely supine resting position is not advised, as you want to remain awake.

NEGATIVITY TREE MEDITATION

(15–20 minutes)

If it is comfortable for you, close your eyes. Otherwise, please soften and lower your gaze. Draw your attention inward. Begin with three deep cleansing breaths. Inhale through your nose and exhale through your mouth with a gentle sigh out.

Transition to inhaling and exhaling through your nose. Begin to breathe evenly, allowing the length of the inhale to match the length of the exhale. For example, inhale four counts, exhale four counts. (3 minutes)

Remember the negative tendency that you wish to dissolve.

Imagine that the seed of that negative tendency has been planted in the left side of your abdomen. It has grown into a massive tree, watered by all the thoughts and actions of this negative tendency. See this tree with its wide trunk of gnarled wood, notice the branches and the fruit that has grown from your negative tendency. Notice how deeply the roots penetrate and how far they reach. (3 minutes)

Place your right hand in front of your face, palm facing you. Fold your index and middle fingers in to touch the pad of the thumb, and extend the ring and pinky finger. You will use the thumb to close off the right nostril and the ring finger to close off the left nostril. Begin by using your thumb to close your right nostril. As you inhale through your left nostril, mentally repeat the mantra for the air element, YAM (pronounced YUM), nine times. Visualize a strong wind uprooting the tree and breaking apart the branches, splintering the wood and smashing the fruit. Hold the breath for three counts. Continue to repeat the mantra YAM and feel the force of the ferocious wind. Next, close off the left nostril with your ring finger and exhale through your right nostril, mentally repeating YAM nine times, continuing to see the wind uprooting and breaking apart the tree. (1 minute)

Now close your right nostril with your thumb and begin to inhale through your left nostril as you repeat the *bija* mantra for the fire element, RAM (pronounced RUM), nine times. Feel, sense, or imagine the tree is being burned. See a blazing fire burning this tree—its roots, branches, and all the fruit. Hold the breath for three counts, counting with the mantra and seeing, feeling, or trusting that the fire is burning the tree. Close off the left nostril and exhale from your right nostril, repeating RAM nine times while continuing to see the tree, fruit, roots, and seeds burning to embers and then ash. Feel all the ash collecting into a small ball. Continue to trust that the entire tree has burned until it is reduced to a small ball of ash. (2 minutes)

Next, close your right nostril and inhale through your left nostril as you repeat the bija mantra for the water element, VAM (pronounced VUM), nine times. Feel, sense, or trust that the rush of water is filling the space, cleansing and washing everything away. Retain the breath for three counts, continuing to repeat the mantra VAM, feeling the fresh purity of water cleansing the space where the tree once was. Close off your left nostril and exhale from the right nostril, mentally repeating VAM nine times as the water continues to wash the space clean. (2 minutes)

Next, close your right nostril and inhale through your left nostril as you repeat the bija mantra for the earth element, LAM (pronounced LUM), nine times. Visualize fresh soil filling in the space where the tree used to be, compacting the fresh soil over the now clean space. Close off your left nostril and exhale from your right nostril while repeating LAM nine times, continuing to see, feel, or sense the fresh soil covering the space. (2 minutes)

Now sense that a beautiful golden ball is emerging from the earth. This golden ball transforms all negative traits. Inhale through both nostrils the bija mantra for ether, HAM (pronounced HUM), nine times. Feel the light expanding as you continue to mentally repeat HAM. Feel the light filling the space of your entire body. (2 minutes)

Eventually this light moves beyond the space of your physical body, filling the space around your body and cocooning you in golden light. Feel that your body, mind, and being are purified. The space outside of your body is purified and filled with golden light. Your negative tendency is purified and repelled by the purity of the golden light that fills and surrounds your body. Feel yourself healed and whole. Allow yourself to be held and cocooned in this light for another two minutes.

Now allow the element of earth to rest at the base of the spine, water in the area of the sacrum, fire at the navel, air at the heart, and space at the throat. All golden light travels to the space of the heart center deep behind the sternum. As the meditation comes to a close, please deepen your breath, gently moving your body in any way that feels supportive for you, and then softly open your eyes, taking in the space around you.

INTENTIONAL PAUSE: FREEWRITING

(3–5 minutes)

Take a few moments to freewrite about your experience with the Negativity Tree Meditation. Do not try to make sense of anything you experienced; write about it without judgment or censorship. Let the words flow from your heart.

Continue this practice for seven to forty consecutive days. If you begin to notice that another trait is being revealed as a subtler expression of the original trait that you chose, you can shift to working with the deeper trait.

SELF-INQUIRY

Consider the following questions:

- How did you experience the practice dissolving your negative tendency? Did you experience sadness, attachment, or resistance in any way?
- Can you pinpoint a time when this negative tendency began? Returning to the Timeline Rewind Practice on page 9 may be helpful to explore this.
- How has this tendency affected your relationships and overall contentment in life?

COMMUNITY CARE

Devote a few moments to consider how this negative trait has affected your ability to create positive relationships within your community. Strengthen the relationships that amplify the qualities that you would like to embody. Notice which relationships you have that cause you to fall back into the patterns of undesirable ways of being. Learn to create boundaries when needed. When you are changing and leaving behind old habits, "show, don't tell"—do your own work and others will notice. When you feel held in a community and appreciate people and family members for being understanding, flexible, and compassionate, let them know.

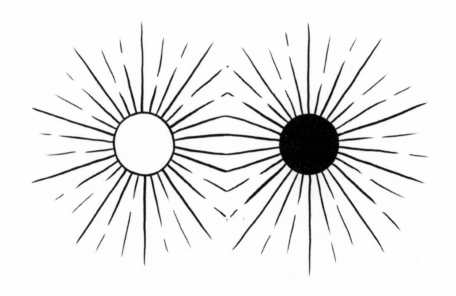

| 3 |

BURNING THE SEEDS OF SORROW— THE POWER OF OPPOSITES

WE ALL EXPERIENCE SOME LEVEL of pain in life, some of us more than others. Pain and sorrow are a part of the human experience. It's a fact that we must accept. When we ignore our pain, it seems to amplify or find other ways to get our attention. First, it may send subtle messages that seem easy to ignore, but eventually the messages will magnify until ignoring them leads to suffering that might be greater than the original pain. We have the capacity to heal from the pain of the past and lessen the effects of future pain if we invite the fullness of our humanness into our spiritual practice. When we plaster a "good vibes only" attitude over our practice, we do ourselves a disservice. When we dive deeper into the smokiness, confusion, and discomfort, we can discover pathways toward our healing.

> Yoga is not a feel-good practice. It is a face-the-truth practice.
> —*Indu Arora*[1]

The second chapter of Patanjali's Yoga Sutras, Sadhana Pada (Chapter of Practice), defines the cause of suffering as avidya (wrong knowledge or ignorance).

The biggest obstacle to our spiritual freedom is mistaking the non-self for the true Self. When we confuse our personality, beliefs, intellect, material possessions, or physical form for who and what we are, we are in ignorance. Remembering who we are requires connecting with the part of ourselves that cannot be taken away, the part of us that is beyond death and decay—that eternal essence that is not confined by time and space. That doesn't mean it's bad to have a body, a personality, material possessions, or opinions. But when we are in touch with a deeper Self, all of what we have is in service to a higher wisdom. True discernment is unclouded by fear, unprocessed pain, and feelings of stuckness. This doesn't mean that you are floating around in some enlightened state, detached from the world. In fact, you may feel your inherent connection to the inner light that is the same light that lights the universe. That moment of connection might last for a moment or a lifetime; when we taste its sweetness, we will forever be changed.

Yogic teachings describe avidya as a veil comprising "seeds of affliction," or kleshas. The kleshas are the root cause of pain and suffering and are divisions of avidya. Avidya is said to be "four footed,"[2] the feet being *asmita* (egoism or I-am-ness), *raga* (attachment), *dvesha* (aversion), and *abinivesha* (fear of death). As the seeds of affliction grow, they give rise to our thoughts and actions and, in turn, those thoughts and actions regenerate and blossom, dropping more seeds that empower the original seeds of affliction. It's a never-ending loop, a field of tangled weeds where the seeds just keep producing poisonous fruit and flowers. It's not enough to just cut down the weeds. Tantric practices help us to burn the seeds until they become inert, diminishing their capacity to produce the results that keep us in pain and suffering.

Yoga Sutra 2:4: avidyā kṣetramuttareṣām prasuptatanuvicchin-nodārāṇām.
Innocence of our divine nature (avidya) creates a fertile field where the seeds of the other four veils take root.
—*Translated by Nischala Joy Devi*[3]

A powerful first step in becoming free from suffering is to acknowledge that at some level we are all in ignorance. We don't know what we don't know. Exploring our personal avidya can create space for powerful insights that help us to find more freedom from discomfort. Please take a moment to read about the *kleshas* below and mindfully answer the accompanying self-inquiry questions. Take breaks when you need to and come back to answer the rest of the questions before moving on. Remember, this practice isn't about judging yourself or others. There are no right or wrong answers, only your truth. This is a practice of inquiry that will help you gain clarity and awaken inner wisdom. In my experience, it is deep inquiry that creates a sliver of space, an interruption in the habitual flow of thoughts and actions that can allow us to make small shifts in our life that lead to more insight and freedom.

AVIDYA

A (not) *vidya* (knowledge) can also be translated as "misperception"; mistaking the body, mind, thoughts, emotions, and feelings for the true Self; confusing things that are noneternal (i.e., our physical bodies) for being eternal. Avidya is always at the root of all the other kleshas. The other four limbs of affliction give avidya the power to run wild and wreak havoc in our lives, keeping us in a cycle of repeating the same mistakes and learning the same lessons over and over. Avidya can take many forms, from believing that we are not worthy of true success in life to believing the earth is flat. We each have our own unique avidya formed by our personal experiences. When we are deep in avidya we might be presented with evidence to support something contrary to what we believe, and instead of pausing to investigate and inquire, we insist on seeing through our coloring on the windshield (*vasana*) that already supports our belief about ourselves and the world. We may even find ourselves shocked by a turn of events because we didn't "see it coming." Avidya has little space or tolerance to allow stillness or contemplation to wash over us and provide a new perspective. Avidya's favorite sayings are "I don't have time or space for practice," "It will never change," and "I already know."

SELF-INQUIRY

Consider the following questions:

- What lesson are you tired of learning?
- What beliefs do you hold that have allowed this pattern to continue?
- How would transforming this pattern change your life?
- Was there ever a time when you didn't see something coming, but in hindsight you realized that all the signs were there? How did the coloring on your windshield prevent you from seeing?

RAGA

Raga is the attachment to what is desirable, and it can manifest as a desire for material wealth, status, power, perfectionism, influence, substances, and accumulation of information. What is desirable for one person may be undesirable for another, so it's important for us to explore what desires we are attached to and how they affect us.

SELF-INQUIRY

Take a moment to list five things that you desire or that you want to make sure that you have in life. We all have a desire for basic needs such as food, clothing, safety, and shelter for ourselves and our loved ones, so create a list that expands beyond this. We are not here to judge ourselves for desiring a designer handbag but to inquire into the nature of our attachments so that we can learn more about ourselves.

1.

2.

3.

4.

5.

As you answer the questions below, notice what emotions or memories arise for you. Raga is strengthened by the pleasure our attachments bring and can easily turn to coveting and greed.

What do you tend to overindulge in and why?

Now, review your list and consider: What would be the result for you if you lost any or all of the things listed? How would it affect you? Emotionally? Spiritually? Practically?

DVESHA

Dvesha is aversion, hate, or repulsion toward what we consider to be undesirable. We all have things that we absolutely want to avoid at all costs. We may avoid certain types of people, foods, places, or experiences in life. These aversions may be related to past traumas and ways to stay safe from harm. It's important to explore these aversions and to discern if we inherited them from relatives or from our own experiences. How do they shape our daily lives and our connection to community and inform intolerance of others?

SELF-INQUIRY

Take a moment to list five things that you have an extreme dislike, aversion, or even hate for.

1.

2.

3.

4.

5.

Now write about *why* you have an aversion to the things you listed. Can you trace these aversions to their roots?

ASMITA

Translated as "I-am-ness" or "egoism," *asmita* is a false sense of identity. It is the belief that the things we know, own, or create are who we are. Asmita relies on the misunderstanding that things that are transient in nature are permanent and that they give us value, hierarchy, and power over others. Asmita denies the interconnectedness that is the nature of reality. This is not say we shouldn't have an ego. We need a healthy ego to exist in the world. But when we overly identify with things that are subject to change, it can lead to instability and the questioning of our value and purpose. I experienced the pull of asmita after closing my yoga studio after ten years. At first I felt the deep loss of the community of amazing students, and as time went on, there were layers of what I perceived as "lost"—the physical space, being a studio owner, being an entrepreneur, being a prominent member of my community. Each loss felt like a part of me was missing. Then it hit me—this is asmita! I had to remind myself that the possessions or titles in life were *expressions* of my true Self; they did not truly define me and were not really "mine" or "me" to begin with. They were all subject to change. Closing my yoga studio only had the power to crush me if I fused the losses with the idea that part of my inherent light was somehow lost along with it. Asmita likes status, power, and control. It is self-centered and believes the ego to be eternal.

SELF-INQUIRY

Take a moment to consider the following questions:

- What accomplishments, titles, or material possessions have you allowed to define you?
- What have you lost in the past that has caused you to question your place in life?
- How are you self-serving? How does this impact your family or community?
- How has ego, excessive pride, or arrogance gotten you into trouble?
- When have you lost something (a job, relationship, possession) only to realize that it set you free?

ABHINIVESHA

Abhinivesha is fear of death, clinging to life, and self-preservation at all costs. There is a whole industry of antiaging, biohacking, and wellness products that exploits our fear of death. Of course, we fear our death and the death of our loved ones. It is natural to want to avoid pain and the chasm of the unknown.

On the spiritual path, we should explore similar questions to what Sri Ramana Maharshi asked: What happens and where do we go when we die? *Who* is dying, and what part of us is beyond aging and decay? The fear of death has many faces. What is it in us that becomes fearful when that new employee stays longer and later in the office than everyone else? If we fear being replaced or overlooked for the next promotion, that can be traced back to abhinivesha. There are countless micro moments in each day in which we experience the fear of death. Trying to deny the fact that every moment we are moving closer and closer to death keeps us in pain. Vyasa's commentary on the Yoga Sutras suggest that we have such an obsession with death because at some level we remember our previous lives and moments of death.[4]

SELF-INQUIRY

Devote a few minutes to considering the following questions:

- What do you fear most about death?
- How many times in this lifetime have you died and been reborn? In how many ways have you had to reinvent yourself?
- Are you living life to the fullest, knowing that one day you will die? What does living life to the fullest mean to you? Are you honoring and spending time with those you love (especially your elders), knowing that they will die one day?

Now take a moment to review all your answers. Notice if there are any recurring themes in your answers.

- Which one of the kleshas is most prevalent in your life right now? Describe how this klesha has caused you discomfort.
- Describe in detail at least one experience of how one of the kleshas has affected you recently.

HOW TO GET FREE

The seeds of affliction (*kleshas*) have four categories of activity: dormant, reduced in force, counteracted, or strongly active. The Yoga Sutras thankfully give us antidotes to help lessen the effect of the kleshas. Through purification practices, the seeking of wisdom, and meditation on the eternal light within, we can begin to find peace. Being present and acknowledging when we feel the pull these veils of ignorance can create the friction of going against the grain of lifelong habits, and that sparks transformation. Cultivating the opposite attitude (*praptipaksha bhavana*) is one of the most direct and intentional practices to lessen the kleshas' hold on us. This power of cultivating the opposite creates an opposing frequency to the dominant klesha, lessening its effect and, with practice, amplifying the opposing attitude until it becomes dominant. This practice helps us clear our mind and become more discerning and peaceful.

> Yoga Sutra 2:33, vitarkabādhane pratiprakṣabhāvanam.
> When doubt or wayward thoughts disturb the cultivation of the yamas and the niyamas, generate the opposite: a counterforce of thoughts, images, or feelings that have the power to uplift, invigorate, inspire, and steady the mind. This is pratipaksha bhavana.
> —*Translated by Reverend Jaganath Carrera*[5]

I leaned on the practice of cultivating the opposites at a very challenging time in my life. I had been betrayed by a romantic partner who was also my business partner. Yes, I ignored all the red flags (*avidya*). There were many entanglements, and the kleshas were in full force. I was attached (*raga*) to my business, which was now dissolving (*abhinivesa*) in front of me. My ego (*asmita*) was wounded, and most of all I was angry (*dvesha*)—angry at how my life had seemingly imploded overnight (*abhinivesha*). We had worked hard to build our business and had big plans (*asmita*). Now they were ruined (*avidya*).

This breakup wasn't as simple as just pressing delete and moving on. Logistically our separation required many phone calls and an endless stream of what then seemed to be unwarranted requests for my time and resources. Every time I saw my ex-partner's name pop up on my phone screen, I would feel the rising heat of anger and annoyance. I could hear myself repeating *my* version of the story, of how I was betrayed, bringing it forward into the present moment and reliving it in real time. Then I remembered a woman I'd met years ago who told me of her partner's betrayal. The story was shocking, and the pain and bitterness was fresh. But when I asked her how long ago it happened, she said, "Ten years ago." Recalling that interaction pushed me into exploring how to heal. I knew I needed a practice to help me. I didn't want to become bitter by holding on to the anger of the past. Then I remembered Yoga Sutra 2:33. I took time to consider what cultivating the opposite of anger would mean. I resisted the answer that arose from my inquiry—compassion. Whew.

I wasn't ready to have in-person conversations or contact with my ex. Everything was still too tender. But I needed to remember that compassion was my healing medicine, so I went into my phone contacts and changed my ex-partner's name to "Be Compassionate." Every time he called or emailed from then on, "Be Compassionate" would pop up on the screen, I would take a deep breath, say his new name out loud, and answer the phone. For the first few weeks, I definitely felt like I was faking it. I was sure the practice wasn't working. I needed to go beyond just the words and feel the vibration of compassion. I started to bring the feeling of compassion into my heart, remembering his troubled childhood and a life of others betraying him. A few weeks after I adapted this new level of compassion, he called, and when I answered he said, "You sound different." I paused and thought to myself, *I AM different.*

I no longer felt the charge that was usually associated with him, his voice, or his name. A spell had been broken. It wasn't a spell he had cast on me but one I had cast on myself—the spell of self-betrayal. I was the one who chose to ignore the red flags, my intuition, and my inner knowing. Committing to compassion created a container of powerful insight. I could see how the seeds of suffering had played their role in my choices and what I thought I knew. My windshield was getting a power wash. The action of cultivating the opposite was the antidote that interrupted the normal flow my habitual thought. This created the space for me to detach from the story. I finally understood a little bit more about the word *vairagya*, which means "dispassion," "detachment," or "transparency." Vairagya is said to be one of the wings of the bird of freedom; the other is practice. I found myself experiencing a little bit more space between what was happening and my reactions. I was neither repulsed by nor attached to my ex-partner, the story of our breakup, or the dissolving of our business. I was in the in-between, a liminal middle ground. I needed to stay in that liminal space, as uncomfortable as it was. I needed to feel everything that was dying so that I could deeply listen to what was waiting to be born within me.

Vairagya gives rise to *viveka*—discriminative wisdom—and in very small ways I began to make better choices, to choose my words more compassionately and truthfully, and to avoid unnecessary conflict and pain. I had been able to find a way through devoted practice (*abyhasa*) and cultivating the opposites to inch my way toward nonattachment, and it felt very freeing. A tiny spoke had been placed in the wheel of karma, protecting me from experiencing the same lesson in my subsequent relationships. This new awareness allowed me to find true love in a devoted, connected, and spiritual partnership with my husband.

SELF-INQUIRY

Consider the following questions:

- What part of you is dying and what part of you is waiting to be born?
- Take a moment to review your answers about which of the kleshas has the strongest hold on you. As you read through them, notice what you feel: excitement, resistance, shame, inspiration, fear? Then as you read through the descriptions, antidotes, and affirmations below, look for clues as to which klesha would serve you best to work with first. Circle anything that resonates with you and make your own notes as you read.

THE ANTIDOTES

Antidotes to our discomfort come in the form of practices, affirmations, and creating space for reflection. When we are ill, we need medicine. Each one of these kleshas is like a poison to our authentic Self. They each have a healing medicine or antidote that counteracts the poison that leads to suffering.

Make no mistake—these kleshas are poisons to our awakening; they keep us asleep to our compassion, insight, and wisdom. It is helpful for us to explore the antidotes and consider what our personal medicine and healing from the kleshas may look like. Weaving the wisdom of antidotes throughout your day is a ritual that requires you to notice when the poison is present. Below I offer suggestions of how to begin creating the inner opening within that will help us to find more ease and peace in life.

Avidya

Avidya, as the underlying current of misunderstanding, pervades all the other kleshas and allows them to thrive, keeping us in a cycle of pain. An antidote to this "absence of knowledge" is of course found through knowledge. But if avidya is also defined as ignorance, we must be aware of how our knowledge is cultivated. In this age of AI-created art, deep fakes, and disinformation it is important to cultivate discernment. Notice if you tend to resonate with things that align with the coloring on your windshield.

Practices: When we are intentionally "cultivating the opposite," we seek every opportunity to practice self-study, learn from wise elders, and be part of communities where we can discuss our experiences and thoughts openly, even when we hold differing opinions. In fact, we may seek to learn from those whose life experiences and beliefs are different from ours and discover where our commonality lies.

Affirmation: May I gain clarity and understanding with deep inquiry and connection.

Asmita

Asmita is the sense of "I-am-ness" that leads to egoism and the feeling that you are your personality, accomplishments, intellect, or status. By cultivating witness consciousness, which helps us to separate our identity from the one who sees, we can begin to lessen the grip of asmita and explore what it means for the persona to be separate from the Self.

Practices: *Pratyahara* (withdrawal of the senses) practices, laya yoga, yoga nidra, heart-centered practices, the study of nature, anonymous donations to organizations, and meditations on death and dying

Affirmation: I am not the doer. I am the one who is eternally at rest.

Raga

Raga is attachment that can manifest as material possessions, creature comforts, relationships, and anything that is pleasurable. Raga is supported by the memory of past pleasures. Work with cultivating the feeling of dispassion by riding the middle way. The concept of dispassion is very nuanced. It's not apathy or a process of forgetting or deleting something or someone from your mind. It is a letting go of gripping. It's an opening of the hand.

Practices: Karma yoga (yoga of selfless service), bhakti yoga (yoga of devotion), decluttering of your personal spaces, committing to acquire only what you need, offering the fruits of your practices for the benefit of others, and the healing of the collective

Affirmation: Not mine. When I remember my true Self, I can share my joy with the world.

Dvesha

The repulsion, loathing, and anger that we feel when dvesha is at play creates resentment, division, oppression, polarization, and violence through our words, thoughts, and actions. It leads to an unwillingness to find common ground, resolution, and mutual understanding. Dvesha is most easily seen when it is directed toward others, but it can also be directed inward where feelings of self-loathing and hatred can overwhelm us.

Practices: Compassion and self-forgiveness practices and prayers, practices that help us be more empathetic and compassionate like the Buddhist practice *tonglen*, self-love practices, practices of deliberation that illuminate cause and effect such as *vichara* or Timeline Rewind (page 9), and writing forgiveness letters and notes of gratitude. Create space for sacred rage.

Affirmation: I have the capacity to be more compassionate. I am worthy of self-forgiveness. I tend to myself with devotion and love. I examine my feelings of aversion with compassion and curiosity. I have the power to pull the poison of hatred from its roots so that I may heal myself.

Abhinivesha

Abhinivesha is the fear of death and our constant companion. We fear the death of our physical self, thinking that is who we are. We fear all of the deaths that can happen to us along the road of life—losing a job, losing reputation, the death of our loved ones, aging, losing our memory, or the ending of our family line or relationships. We can begin to inquire into our fear of death by contemplating: Is the physical body needed for the true Self to exist?

Practices: Yoga nidra, guided savasana (see page 125), restorative yoga, sound healing, inner-light meditations (see page 146), death practices (see pages 113–14), and being present and supportive for someone going through the dying process

Affirmations: My love and inner light are eternal. May I remember the part of me that was there when the universe was created.

CULTIVATING OPPOSITES RITUAL

Doing practices to free yourself from pain and suffering is the practice of Self-devotion. Tending to the Self is part of what is required for our collective healing to occur. When we know what heals us, we can share that healing with our community. Take a moment to create an altar of Self-devotion. At first this may seem self-indulgent. But it is necessary to begin to own the ways in which you currently don't take care of yourself and to begin a new way of tending not just to your outer body but to your inner Self.

Begin with a simple candle, a seed, and a piece of paper. Choose a seed intentionally. Something that has significance to you, that works with your growing season and climate, and that can be grown indoors.

Take a moment to read the care instructions for your future plant.

Choose a small sunlit corner to place your altar.

Before you plant your seed, hold it between your hands. Remember the klesha you chose to work with and its antidote. Offer yourself a blessing.

Place the candle on the altar. On a small piece of paper, write the affirmation that is an antidote to the klesha you have decided to work on. You can use the affirmation suggested above or you can create your own.

Place your affirmation on the table. Consider framing it or making a creative piece of art.

Each day, light your candle, water your seed, and repeat your affirmation.

The candle flame represents the light of your true Self.

The affirmation represents the promise you have made to yourself to tend to Self-devotion and the reminder of the medicine needed to heal.

Your daily watering is a reminder of how to tend with love and devotion.

Repetition of the affirmation is creating new neural pathways in the brain, renewing the desire for sacred remembrance and the desire to know your true Self. Notice as you move through the day when you feel the klesha arising. Pause, receive a few breaths, and repeat the affirmation, either silently or out loud. Practice for a minimum of forty days.

As you continue to tend to this plant, devote some time every few weeks to journal about what you have observed and learned from the practice. How can you apply what you have learned to your relationship with yourself and others?

COMMUNITY CARE

Observe in group settings where the kleshas might be at play. Practice non-judgment, nonviolent communication, and detachment. Learn to observe and ask yourself: *What do I see? What do I feel? What have I learned?*[6] Notice what your opinions and reactions are rooted in. Learn to listen and practice empathy. This will help you to develop discernment. Imagine ways to bring antidotes to conversations. Consider asking questions that may bring more awareness and insight. Create boundaries when needed.

This will take practice and embodiment derived from your own practices with cultivating opposites. Don't rush the process. When in doubt, compassion is always the way.

OBSERVING RESISTANCE AND THE NINE FORMIDABLE OBSTACLES

On every spiritual journey, we will find resistance to our expansion in the form of obstacles. Stumbling blocks are to be expected; learning to move through resistance often empowers our devotion to practice, expands our capacity, and fortifies our resilience. When we understand what obstacles consistently emerge for us, we become aware of our patterns and can begin the work to set ourselves free.

The Yoga Sutras speak directly to nine specific obstacles known as the *antarayas* (impediments or obstacles) in Yoga Sutra 1: 30:

yādhi styāna saṁśaya pramāda-ālasya-avirati bhrāntidarśana-alabdha-bhūmikatva-anavasthitatvāni citta-vikṣepāḥ te antarāyāḥ

The obstacles are considered "nine disruptive forms of consciousness" that prevent us from maintaining mental clarity.[7] They are disease, dullness, doubt, carelessness, sloth, over-externalizing the senses, delusion, not understanding the goal of yoga, and instability.

Devote a few minutes to the exploring list of obstacles below. Note which obstacles feel the most relevant and present currently. Make notes in your journal on how they manifest in your life and practice.

1. Sickness or dis-ease (*vyadhi*) are physical ailments or discomfort that prevent you from practicing. Remember how to make practices

accessible for yourself and offer yourself grace. Grace is a form of practice.

2. Procrastination or mental dullness (*styana*) can happen when we neglect our mental health or experience mental lethargy.

3. Doubt (*samshaya*) is the feeling that it can't be done or it won't be done because something is lacking within us. We doubt the process, our progress, and ourselves. We lack faith, which may cause indecision and stuckness in our practice.

4. Carelessness (*pramada*) is a form of consciousness where we are neglectful, inconsistent, and lacking foresight. We may learn the same lessons repeatedly because we are forgetful, sloppy, and "going through the motions" in our practices, especially if we forget to practice the eight limbs of yoga.[8]

5. Sloth (*alasya*) is excess inertia that may cause an inability to feel motivated and inspired.

6. Over-externalizing the senses (*avirati*) is the inability to withdraw the senses inward, practice detachment, or honor the need for a place of rest and sanctuary. We misplace our attention on the external world when we need to turn inward. Instead, there may be an insatiable craving to explore the world of the senses, which pulls us away from our practices.

7. Delusion (*brantidarsana*) is confusion about the goal of practice.

8. Losing traction (*alabdha-bhumikatva*) is not understanding the goal of practice and lacking the capacity to remain aligned with the goal because we doubt we can even succeed.

9. Instability (*anavashitava*) is lacking groundedness, the ability to cultivate stillness and claim your place in the world.

This list of disturbances is something that we all experience to some degree at different times in life. The purpose of sharing this sutra is not for us to judge ourselves but for us to become aware of how we may be experiencing a holding pattern as we do the deeper work. The Yoga Sutras give us signs to look out for that may provide clues to figuring out if what we are experiencing is one of the nine obstacles. Those signs are mental discomfort, negative thinking, and difficulty controlling our breath. These are all mentioned in the following sutra, 1:31.

Practice: Devote some time to noticing how and when these obstacles show up for you in real time. When you experience one of the nine arising, pause and either write a few notes about it or take a few deep breaths if you are short on time. Pausing with presence will help you interrupt the flow of disturbances and increase your awareness. Recommitting to a consistent practice rooted in devotion and daily remembrance of the Divine within you helps soften the effects of the antarayas.

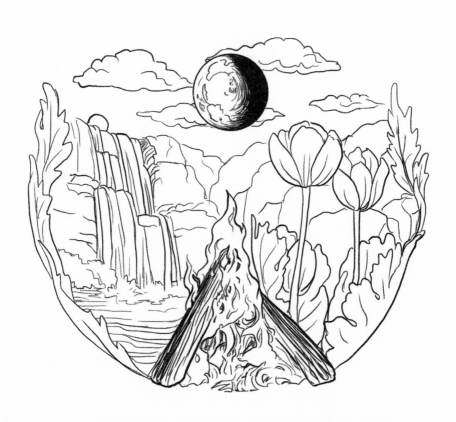

| 4 |

AWAKENING OUR
ELEMENTAL NATURE

Dear Mother,

Please take me in your arms and hold me.

Remind me that it is from you that I have come and will return.

It helps me to have the courage to lay down and imagine
     dissolving into the infinite.

Then I can truly rest.

Please guide my journey with your morning light, stars, and moon.

This helps me to remember that I am lit from within.

May your sacred waters purify me, so I can ride the ebbs and
     flows of life with discernment and clarity.

Your graceful love and abundance is unconditional.

Thank you.

Your power can be fierce, and this teaches me respect.

May I always remember to cherish, honor, and protect you.

—Tracee Stanley

I HAD MY FIRST INSIGHT that I was something more than the gross mass of my physical body and personality early one summer in the hours before sunrise in 1995. I was sitting on my balcony in a small neighborhood in Cape Town, South Africa. Tamboerskloof is nestled in the foothills of Lion's Head and Signal Hill mountains; from my balcony, I had a view of the majestic Table Mountain. That morning she was covered with a flowing "tablecloth" of clouds pouring over her edges. The sun was just about to rise, and as I sat on that balcony in silence, everything seemed perfectly still. There was nowhere to go and nothing to do. I was content with submerging myself in the beauty that surrounded me. Having spent the last several years living in metropolitan cities around the world, I could not remember when I had experienced such stillness. I was in awe of how the clouds looked like smoke, moonlight, and water flowing together in a beautiful and seductive dance to slowly reveal the mountain. As the clouds dissolved in the stillness, it seemed that all my problems, worries, and thoughts dissolved along with them. Nothing existed except the flow of the clouds. For the first time, I was awake to the experience of presence. I wasn't intentionally meditating. I was fully immersed in being.

I felt spacious and free. I could sense what seemed like long gaps of nothingness. In a moment of what I can only describe as grace, I felt myself let go of gripping. I experienced a vibration. It felt like my whole body was vibrating and pulsing. I remained still and surrendered into the beauty, and then a sense came over me that was a knowing. I felt like every important question I had was answered. It seemed to last forever, as if time stood still. Soon the sun was rising, the birds were chirping, and I became aware that something profound had happened, something I could not name. I had gone somewhere beyond time; it felt like home from a long, long time ago. My body was still vibrating. I was supercharged. Something inside of me had been revealed. This wasn't something that happened to me. It was me. My mind began trying to make sense of what had happened, but it had nothing to compare it to. What I know now is that I experienced a moment of spontaneous meditation that allowed a part of me that was hidden to briefly emerge as a vibration of utter peace, tranquility, and knowing. I experienced my core frequency, a vibration of the me without the labels, the worries, and the fears. For someone who had never meditated before, this was a revelatory experience and was the moment that led me to the path of yoga.

This meditative moment of spacious awareness didn't require flexibility or the physical prowess that we have been led to believe are the most important aspects of yoga. I didn't need a technique; I had this experience of deep stillness and peace by simply observing nature with awe and gratitude. Layers had been peeled back to reveal a frequency underlying everything and I felt connected to everything around me.

INTENTIONAL PAUSE: REMEMBERING AWE

Remember a time when you experienced awe, stillness, or presence. It could have happened while being in nature, having a great run, painting, singing, dancing, giving birth, hiking, jumping into a cold river, meditating, making love, enjoying the opera, or experiencing the moments between sleeping and waking. Devote a few minutes to freewriting about the experience, how you felt, where you were, what you were doing, and *why* it was so memorable.

THE NATURE WITHIN

There is a world of nature around us that holds the key to helping us remember who we are. I use the word *remember* because memory (*smirti*) is one of the keys to knowing our true Self. Even though I had a powerful experience in the awe of Table Mountain, as time went by, I began to forget the fullness of the experience.

One of the biggest illusions of the ego-self is that we are separate from nature. We are nature; there is no separation. Tantric teachings and many wisdom traditions tell us that we are nature, and the same elements that are present in nature are also inside of us. Everything is made up of five basic elements, known as the *panchamahabhutas* (five great elements): earth (*prithvi*), water (*jala*), fire (*tejas*), wind (*vayu*), and ether or space (*akasha*). If the matter that is found in the universe is also found inside our bodies; we each can think about our body as a microcosm of the larger macro universe. When we consider this, we begin to understand how what we do in the outer world affects our personal inner world and vice versa. If we deplete the earth of resources, we will feel depleted. If we neglect to heal our broken hearts, the collective will be brokenhearted. If we promote divisiveness and separation, we will never feel whole. Remembering the nature of our true Self is what we need to begin recollecting the broken pieces of this world.

The suggestion of "nature," however, does not bring up images of peaceful waterfalls, majestic mountains, and awe for everyone. We must acknowledge the trauma that may live in our DNA and memories that relate to the idea of being immersed in nature. When growing up, I was told not to go into the woods near my house. The "woods" held some unseen danger, and this idea was reinforced by many fairy tales, like "Little Red Riding Hood" and "Hansel and Gretel." I remember seeing the movie *Roots* and watching enslaved people running for their lives through the deep forest and being captured there. Nature was not a safe place until I began to consciously reclaim its presence within *me*.

I still don't go hiking on "private land" without permission, even when others say, "Oh, I hike here all the time." We all may be storing some intergenerational trauma of ancestors. If our people have been stolen, "relocated," or forced to flee from their ancestral lands, we can feel separated from nature— disconnected from a deep source of our power, lineage, ancestral foods, healing practices, and stories. It is unwise to ignore the possible effects of colonization and the traumas you may have internalized or inherited that may affect your ability to cultivate a reciprocal relationship with nature that is inherent to who you are. I have always been a strong swimmer, but I was very afraid of the deep ocean even though I had spent a lot of time on our family boat growing up. I had no reason to be fearful of drowning in the ocean. Could it have been intergenerational trauma from the Middle Passage when countless enslaved African people were thrown overboard? The psychologist Mariel Buqué says that for Black people, water represents "one of the largest collective traumas we have experienced in the Western Hemisphere."[1] It is important for us to explore our relationship with nature as it relates to the history of our ancestors and their indigenous homelands.

INTENTIONAL PAUSE: SELF-INQUIRY

Take a moment to consider your relationship with nature and what she means to you.

- Recall a time when you felt a deep connection with the natural environment around you. Describe in detail where you were, how old you were, and what you experienced.
- What scares you most about being in nature?
- Who in your life had a deep respect for nature and shared their love with you? How did they share? What connection do you have to your ancestral homeland?
- Have you ever felt unsafe in nature? If so, why?

The exploration of nature and its cycles is a gateway to self-understanding. The more present we are to the cycles of nature—the transitions of seasons; the reality of birth, death, and rebirth, which includes the transitions of the day—the more we learn about the reality of life and forge an interconnectedness to nature that guides us with harmony, acceptance, and respect of the natural world. When we feel ourselves as nature, we heal ourselves from one of the most the massive forgettings of our times. This global amnesia and disconnection from nature have already produced consequences that will affect generations to come in unimaginable ways.

Many wisdom traditions honor and recognize five elements as essential to the spiritual understanding of who we are.[2] Different elements are honored in various traditions. In the yogic traditions, the main elements that are explored are earth, water, fire, air, and ether or space. These elements are associated with the chakra system that is part of our subtle anatomy. The chakras hold many of the impressions and imprints of our life. Connecting with these elements help us to progress in understanding ourselves from the most gross aspects to the subtlest.

Ayurveda teaches that the body is associated with the elements. For example, the feet to the thighs is associated with the earth—not only are they the heaviest parts of our body, the feet and legs are most often in relationship with the earth. This is an especially important understanding in practices of laya yoga (the yoga of dissolution), such as yoga nidra. It is the combination of these elements that creates the *doshas*, or "three humors": vata (air and ether), pitta (fire and water), and kapha (earth and water).

The Dagara tribe in West Africa honors earth, water, fire, mineral, and nature itself as the elements. Japanese cultures honor the element of wood, which relates to the forests. Native American peoples consider each element and living being of the earth a relative and teacher, depending on the tribe. Traditional Chinese Medicine associates the elements with various organs in the body. Doing some research on how your culture understands and honors the elements is a way to connect with the ancestral wisdom within you.

We will explore the following elements as we continue to journey together through the rest of the book. Take some time to consider each of these aspects of nature and freewrite about any insights you have about them. I've added some words and suggestions for connection practices to inspire contemplation of the multidimensionality of these elements and their many manifestations throughout your life. The practices in bold can be found in "Additional Practices" at the back of the book. I recommend committing to doing each one of these practices over the next year, with time spent freewriting afterward. Give yourself grace as you explore each element. If you are attracted to other elements that do not appear on this list, find intuitive ways to honor and awaken to them.

	Manifestations	Qualities	Practices
Earth	The Great Mother, fertility, soil, foundation, home, abundance, beauty	Supportive, grounded, rooted, nurturing, generative, regenerative, giving, blessing, inclusive, belonging	Earthing, walking barefoot on the ground, **Earth honoring practices** (see pages 57–63)
Water	Ocean, rivers, tributaries, rain	Flowing, purifying, hydrating, life-sustaining, full of momentum, emotional, yielding, all-conquering	Soaking in hot springs, float tanks, ritual baths, observing the ocean waves, anointing
Air	Breath, life, wind	Movement, change, flexibility, trust in the unseen, circulation	**Pranayama** (page 161), breathwork
Fire	Digestion, transformation, combustion, processing, willpower, *sankalpa* (heartfelt desire), alchemy	Heating, creativity, alchemy	Fire ceremony, *agni sara*, observing the movement of wildfire and fire weather, building an internal fire
Ether/ Space	Spirit, container, unlimited potentiality, infinity, the celestial	Vast, open, spacious, expansive, welcoming, multidimensional	Yoga nidra, meditation, learning to hold sacred space
Mineral	Bones, stone, gems, crystal, memory, deeper knowledge, wisdom	Ancestral, resourceful, deep, wise	Ancestor rituals (see pages 120–130), memory exercises, meditating with or on rock formations in energetically charged sites, meditating with crystals
Nature	Birth, death, rebirth, transmutation, seasons, magic	Cyclical, fierce, powerful, abundant, supernatural, complex, interconnected	Seasonal rituals, gardening, caregiving for an ill or dying person, honoring death (see page 113), celebrating life, observing one spot in nature daily for a season, observing transitions

INTENTIONAL PAUSE: SELF-INQUIRY

Now consider the following questions:

- Which of these elements do you feel the most connected to and why? Describe an experience of profound connection.
- Which of the elements do you understand the least? Which element feels most foreign to you?

DATTATREYA GURUS

One of my favorite stories in the Vedic teachings is about the young sage Dattatreya. Dattatreya was said to be an incarnation of Vishnu, Bramha, and Shiva in one body. He came to earth to deliver wisdom and truth in a dark time. When Dattatreya was a young boy, a king recognized his radiance and was curious to know how it was that he was enlightened at such a young age. He wanted to know the name of his guru. Dattatreya responded that he had twenty-four gurus. They were: Mother Earth, water, fire, wind, space, moon, sun, flock of pigeons, python, ocean, moth, bumblebee, elephant, ant, fish, courtesan, arrow maker, infant/playful child, deer, bird of prey, maiden, serpent, spider, and worm. Each one of these aspects of nature provided a portal for enlightenment and wisdom. Over the last two decades I have been fortunate enough to live close to nature in the mountains. The first things I like to do when I am in a new home is to learn about the indigenous people of the land and then I make an ongoing list of all of the animals that I share the land with. It usually takes several weeks or sometimes seasons to observe who else is around. Recently I moved to a small village in northern New Mexico. Shortly after we moved into the house I observed a family of deer traversing a game trail right outside my bedroom porch. I would watch them every morning as they grazed on the vegetation and soon began to recognize some of the members of the herd. As the season began to transition toward autumn, the deer came to eat from the crabapple tree growing in front of the house. I watched as they effortlessly jumped over the fence to eat the fruit. I thought about Dattatreya and what I could learn from these beautiful animals. And then one day I locked eyes with one of the doe, we eye-gazed for nearly three minutes before the other deer hurried her along. She was peaceful and alert, curious and loving. She seemed to know that I had been watching for months. What I learned from her that day was that an unconditional loving gaze can connect two hearts.

NATURE AWARENESS RITUAL

Self-paced

Take time to consider your environment, whether you live deep in nature or in the city. Which of Dattatreya's gurus are present? Make a list of all the animals, insects, and elements that are present and keep adding to it. Set ten minutes aside, one day a week, to observe these gurus in their natural environment. What do you notice according to the season, weather, or time of day? What lessons does the nature around you have to offer? If you have the space, consider planting a small garden and observe the plants for their full life cycle. After each nature awareness practice, devote five minutes to journaling or freewriting about what you learned.

AS ABOVE, SO BELOW MEDITATION

10–15 minutes

You can find audio of this practice at www.shambhala.com/TheLuminousSelf Practices.

The Shiva Samhita states, "As it is in the macrocosm, so it is in the microcosm."[3] Remember that there is a universe inside of you. If you want to experience change, you can begin by becoming aware of your inner universe. You can connect with the power vortexes within you, purify your inner elements, and balance your solar and lunar qualities. The following meditation is a journey through your inner universe.

Please find a supportive and comfortable meditative shape. Begin to notice the natural flow of the breath. Notice the quality of the mind and the quality of the breath and how the two reflect each other. (1 minute)

Begin to gently shape the breath by allowing it to become smooth, quiet, and equal lengths on inhale and exhale. (2 minutes)

Remember that there is a whole universe inside of you. As above, so below. Become aware of lunar energy. Inhale through the left nostril and exhale through the right. No mudra is needed; only the power of your mind. Once again, inhale through the left nostril and exhale through the right. Feel, sense, or trust the presence of a cooling lunar quality that is nurturing, soothing, healing, and the color of moonlight. (10 breaths)

Contemplate the qualities of solar energy as you shift attention to the right nostril. Inhale through the right nostril and exhale through the left. Notice the heating qualities of strength, dynamism, and vitality. Inhale through the right nostril and exhale through the left. (10 breaths)

Feel a balancing of solar and lunar energy. Sense that you have been purified by the heating qualities of the sun and equally purified by the healing nectar of the moon.

Gently begin to breathe in through both nostrils and out through both nostrils. Continue to feel the breath as smooth, quiet, and even. Let your attention rest inside the central axis of your body, the spine. Sense the spine as a river of light flowing upward. (10 breaths)

Feel the presence of the energy centers, chakras resting inside the spine as islands. Each island is a vortex of power.

Bring awareness to the base of the spine, to the first chakra. Connect with the element of earth and the quality of patience.

Bring awareness to the next island located in the sacrum region. Connect with the element of water and the quality of purity.

Bring awareness to the next island located in the region of the navel center. Connect with the element of fire and the quality of radiance.

Travel upward to the next island located at the region of the heart. Connect with the element of air and the quality of contentment.

Continue to travel upward to the island in the throat center. Connect with the element of ether or space and the quality of unity.

Bring awareness to the island in the space between the eyebrows, a place beyond the elements. Connect with the power of the qualities of divine communication and discernment.

Let attention rise to the crown center, connecting to Divine Consciousness and oneness.

Imagine all the rivers, stars, and galaxies within your body. Experience your entire body and the space around your body as a universe. Seeing. Feeling. Trusting. Experience yourself as the universe. (2–5 minutes)

When you are ready to complete the meditation, come back slowly. Devote several minutes to freewriting, journaling, or transcribing your experience of the practice.

CONNECTED ROOTS MEDITATION

(10–15 minutes)

Please find a comfortable meditation shape and either close your eyes or soften your gaze. As you settle in, begin to notice your body breathing. As your body receives an inhale, your navel rises; as your body releases an exhale, your navel falls. Continue to watch the rise and fall of your navel for ten breaths.

Begin to notice the flow of breath moving through your left nostril. Feel as though all of your breath can move in through your left nostril and out through your right nostril. You do not need to use any mudras or fingers, just the power of your mind. Where your mind goes, energy flows. In through the right and out through the left. Continue to alternate the flow of breath between your nostrils. (2 minutes)

Breathe in through both nostrils and out through both. (10 times)

Begin to feel your spine as the central axis of your body. Sense the space to the right of your spine, to the left of your spine, behind your spine, and in front of your spine. Now sense the space inside your spine and begin to feel a flow of energy or vibration moving from the base of your spine to your third-eye point as you inhale, and from the third-eye point to the base of your spine as you exhale.

Sense that your spine is like a tree trunk. Each time you exhale, feel and sense the roots of the tree growing down deep into the earth. On the inhale, awareness rises from the roots to your third-eye point. Each time your body exhales, the roots of the tree grow deeper; feel them connecting with other root systems, notice the nourishment and stability that arises from these connected roots. Sense how these roots connect the other trees in a great forest. Feel yourself as the interconnected tapestry of not only roots but forest canopy, home to many species of birds, animals, plants, and fungi. Feel yourself nourished and whole, supported by community and nature. (5 minutes)

Begin to breathe deeply and slowly bring yourself back by allowing your eyes to flutter open, letting the light filter in. Devote five minutes to freewriting. After you have finished writing, spend a few moments offering your gratitude to the earth, perhaps by watering the nearest tree or saying a simple prayer of gratitude.

COMMUNITY CARE

Sharing an experience in nature for a day can be a healing and restorative practice. Start conversations with members of your community about their relationship with nature. Many times, being afraid of nature can be a source of shame or even humor. There are countless horror movies with a plot that begins with being lost or stranded in the woods. It's no wonder we have a collective fear of being alone in nature. Share your experiences and notice where you have commonalities. Take a group of friends, family, or elders for a day of picnicking in the forest, by a lake, walking in nature, or laying on the earth or stargazing at night. Normalize the activity of spending time in nature and spacious silence, without devices and distractions, to realign. Sit together and practice the Connected Roots Meditation. Feel yourselves as members of the great forest. Share your insights and inspirations afterward.

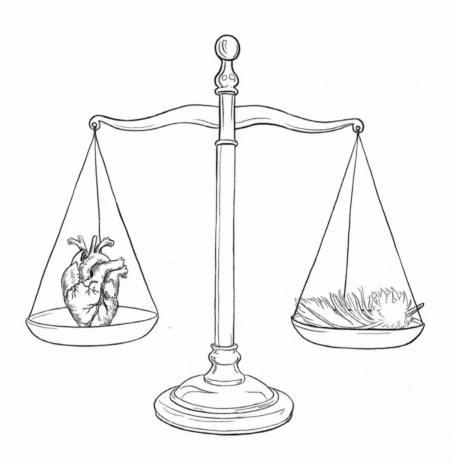

| 5 |

RECOLLECTION AND
RECONCILIATION

OUR ABILITY TO RECALL what is essential is more fragile now than ever. We have so many distractions. I am not referring to the kind of distraction that accompanies stress, overwhelm, hormonal changes, or memory loss due to aging. We, as a culture, are willfully choosing not to remember. The smartphone[1] erased our desire to remember phone numbers, addresses, or directions. Media outlets compete for our attention in a never-ending cycle of news and clickbait. The speed at which we scroll for information leaves us unable to digest and retain what we are consuming. We do not hold on to important information, especially if we know it can easily be found on the internet or our smartphones. We are outsourcing special memories and moments of awe to our photo libraries. We spend our time documenting our lives like photojournalists instead of being present in the moment and the emotions that arise in real time. If it's not stored in our phone, it didn't happen. This forgetting is what scientists call "digital amnesia"—using our devices to store data instead of our long-term memory.[2] We are more distracted and forgetful than ever. Young and old, it's affecting us all. And the COVID-19 pandemic that began in 2020 may have only increased digital amnesia.

Yogic philosophers spoke about the importance of memory. The Sanskrit word *smriti* comes from the root word *samra* and can be translated as "that which is remembered." Smriti is both an essential part of practice and an effect of devoted practice. Smriti is one of the paths to spiritual liberation and is more than the remembering of facts, information, or teachings. Yoga Sutra 1:20 names smriti as one of the five methods to reach samadhi (enlightenment) the others being faith, inner strength, insight, and mental focus.

One of the twenty-five paths named in the *Nyaya Sutras* that is said to help reclaim and awaken memory is the practice of viyoga.[3] Viyoga refers to the act of separating—the opposite of yoga, of which the root word, *yuj*, means "union." As it relates to memory, viyoga asks us to remember what has caused us pain and what has caused us pleasure. Remembering what has caused us pain may help us avoid repeating the same lessons over and over. Recognizing what is considered unpleasant may also allow us to reframe experiences and see new things that are layered underneath what was considered undesirable. In this way, it is possible to see where pain has also made us stronger, wiser, more insightful, and more compassionate. This can also help us understand where there may be trauma, unprocessed emotions, and healing that requires the support of a great therapist.

INTENTIONAL PAUSE: REVIEW AND REFLECT

In the first three chapters, we explored how we are shaped by the imprints of life that we consider good, bad, or neutral. Take a few moments to review your reflections on the self-inquiry questions from chapters 1–4.

- What, if anything, stands out to you as you reread your reflections and journaling from the previous chapters?
- Did you notice any recurring themes or things that surprised you?
- Did you write about anything that you didn't remember writing about?

Yoga practices can help us reassemble ourselves by reclaiming the forgotten parts of ourselves, our experiences, and life lessons. This kind of intentional remembering fosters integrating, assimilating, and processing. It allows us to review our lives and let go of what feels stagnant by churning and witnessing it as food for our evolution. What is left is then nourishing and sustaining instead of depleting. Devote a few moments to explore the following inquiries:

- What part of your essential Self are you ready to reclaim?
- Which of your unique gifts, talents, and inner beauty have you forgotten or neglected?
- How are you careless with the most sacred parts of yourself and your life?

Community Care

Make an effort to remember what is sacred, painful, and important to others. Learn how to hold space for people without needing to know more than they are willing to share. Resist the urge to gossip about or judge whatever is shared with you. Learn to understand when silence is healing, even in a room full of people. We all want to be seen, heard, and felt. When we are truly seen by others, the heart has a healing resonance. Create opportunities in your communities to practice heartfelt conversations that are not based on "What can you do for me?" or "How can I uplevel myself by being in relationship with this person?" Notice when relationships, friendships, or communities may be holding a transactional quality; find ways to shift into being in aligned and loving relationships.

FORGIVENESS IS FREEDOM

A forgiving heart knows the art of liberation.

—John O'Donohue[4]

Forgiveness is one of the most potent tools of healing. Forgiveness gives us opportunities to reconcile with other people and with ourselves. The word *reconcile* refers to the bringing back together of things. When we embrace forgiveness, we allow ourselves to remember our wholeness.

We can begin to transform our relationship to forgiveness by embracing self-forgiveness. Choosing to forgive is an act of compassion toward yourself. That said, forgiveness isn't easy. It's not as simple as saying, "I choose to forgive," especially when we are dealing with the effects of trauma or post-traumatic stress disorder (PTSD). The important thing to remember is that forgiveness does not require the participation of anyone but yourself. It is an internal process between you and your own heart. You get to decide when and if you are ready and what forgiveness means to you. "I am deeply anchored in my opinion that we do not owe anyone who has harmed us our forgiveness," says Zahabiyah Yamasaki, the director of Transcending Sexual Trauma through Yoga. "We are, however, *worthy of our own forgiveness* for all the ways we may have internalized shame or blame that was never ours to carry." Self-forgiveness is a practice that takes time and may require the support of a skilled therapist or spiritual mentor. Yamasaki offers that "self-forgiveness in the healing journey might look like forgiving yourself for the years spent in survival mode—operating with coping mechanisms that kept you safe but perhaps made it hard to rest. Self-forgiveness might look like upholding and honoring a boundary that you used to let slide. Self-forgiveness might look like saying no to honor your capacity, even when you want to say yes. Self-forgiveness might be finally believing you are truly and deeply enough just as you are."[5]

Self-forgiveness is often the first step in the journey of healing. In the following section, you will find practices and inquiries to help facilitate forgiveness. Take your time to move through them. If you approach any of these practices and receive a hard intuitive *no*, trust yourself and only work with what feels right for you in your own time. If you feel difficult emotions arise at any point in the practices below, take as much time as you need to pause, freewrite, go outside, shake your body, or do the jibba jabba practice (page 11) and return if and when and if you are called to continue. If something doesn't feel right for you, skip it.

SELF-FORGIVENESS RITUAL

Follow these eight steps to creating your letter, adding any other intuitive elements that you find supportive and healing.

1. Clear space and time to write your forgiveness letter. Set up a rest nest for yourself to be able to rest in either while you write it or to rest in afterward. Bring anything into the space that would be comforting: a cup of hot tea, soothing music, sacred smokes, or comfy blankets. Make sure those who you may share space with know that you are in ritual space and shouldn't be disturbed.

2. In your letter, describe the situation that you want to offer yourself forgiveness for.

3. Describe how this situation affected you.

4. Describe why it is that you have decided to offer yourself forgiveness at this time.

5. Take breaks when you need to and ask for support if needed.

6. Describe your hopes, desires, and new possibilities that you imagine will come to fruition from this offering of self-forgiveness.

7. Create a sacred fire to burn the letter if you choose or you can keep it on your altar as a sacred reminder. Create a piece of art or a poem inspired by your letter.

8. If you decide to burn the letter, you can save the ashes and offer them to your compost heap, bury them, or release them in a body of water.

INTENTIONAL PAUSE: FORGIVENESS CONTEMPLATION

Devote some time to contemplating and answering the following questions. Give yourself spaciousness to write and reflect. I suggest fifteen to thirty minutes.

- Is there any person whom you feel anger or resentment toward? Any situation? Write about a few instances and include a few where you feel ready to forgive.
- Decide if you are ready to forgive a situation or person that has caused you pain. Pause here and ask yourself what circumstances would need to be present for you to forgive. Is the situation too fresh?
- Does this situation or person deserve your forgiveness? What is best for *your* healing?
- What does it look like for you to hold a sacred boundary, protect your heart, and take your time in the process of healing? Be honest with your answers and let go of any judgment around your responses.

TONGLEN

The word *tonglen* comes from two words: *tong* means "giving" or "sending," and *len* means "receiving" or "taking." Tonglen is also known as exchanging the self with the other. I first encountered this practice in 2000 when I read Pema Chödrön's seminal book *When Things Fall Apart*. I had experienced a heartbreak and tried to distract myself with a yoga retreat to Maui. I picked up this book merely because of the title, and I found the practice of tonglen. The amount of resistance I had to practicing tonglen when I first read about it gave me the signal that I needed to pause and feel into whether it was right for me and whether I was ready to forgive. It has been a transformative practice for me in my life. I am forever grateful that I have been permitted to offer tonglen here.

TONGLEN PRACTICE

When you do tonglen as a formal meditation practice, it has four stages:

1. Rest your mind briefly in a state of openness or stillness for a second or two. This stage is traditionally called flashing on absolute *bodhichitta*, or suddenly opening to basic spaciousness and clarity.

2. Work with texture. Breathe in a feeling of hot, dark, and heavy—a sense of claustrophobia—and breathe out a feeling of cool, bright, and light—a sense of freshness. Breathe in completely, through all the pores of your body, and breathe out completely, radiating through all the pores of your body. Continue this until the practice synchronizes with your in- and out-breaths.

3. Work with a personal situation—any painful situation that's real to you. Traditionally you begin by doing tonglen for someone you care about and wish to help. However, as I described, if you are stuck, you can do the practice for the pain you are feeling and simultaneously for all those just like you who feel that kind of suffering. For instance, if you are feeling inadequate, you breathe that in for yourself and all the others in the same boat, and you send out confidence and adequacy or relief in any form you wish.

4. Finally, make the taking in and sending out bigger. If you are doing tonglen for someone you love, extend it out to those who are in the same situation as your friend. If you are doing tonglen for someone you see on television or on the street, do it for all the others in the same boat. Make it bigger than just that one person. If you are doing tonglen for all those who are feeling the anger, fear, or whatever that you are trapped in, maybe that's big enough. But you could go further in all these cases. You could do tonglen for people you consider to be your enemies—those who hurt you or hurt others. Do tonglen for them, thinking of them as having the same confusion and stuckness as your

friend or yourself. Breathe in their pain and send them relief. Tonglen can extend infinitely. As you do the practice, gradually, over time, your compassion naturally expands and so does your realization that things are not as solid as you thought. As you do this practice, gradually at your own pace, you will be surprised to find yourself more and more able to be there for others even in what used to seem like impossible situations.

Note: When you do tonglen on the spot, simply breathe in and breathe out, taking in pain and sending out spaciousness and relief.

COMMUNION OF THE HIGHER SELVES PRACTICE
(approx. 15 minutes)

This meditation asks us to connect our higher mind, highest Self, or buddhi (discernment). When we connect to this place within, we remember our multidimensionality. The higher mind, or buddhi, is a place within us that knows. It is beyond the place of right and wrong, good and bad. It doesn't rely on the storehouse of memories or our ego for its direction. It takes its direction from the light of the soul. If we can imagine our higher Self having a meeting with another person's higher Self, we may be able leave blame behind and have a new perspective on the situation.

Find a quiet and comfortable place to practice. This practice is generally done sitting up but can also be practiced lying down. Find an easeful meditation posture or reclined position. Allow your back to be supported by bolsters, a chair, a wall, or a bed—whichever is most comfortable for you.

Begin by witnessing your body breathing in and out. Let go of the desire to "take" a breath; soften and allow the breath to be received. (5 breaths)

Let your attention settle on your abdomen and observe how your belly expands and contracts as your breath moves in and out of your body. (10 breaths)

Now move your awareness upward to rest at your heart center. Begin to feel as though your breath is moving in and out through your heart center. Feel connected to the part of yourself that has an inner knowing, a higher intelligence. This part of you knows both the cause and the cure of pain. Feel the expansiveness that accompanies the connection to your higher Self. Imagine, feel, or visualize your highest Self filled with and surrounded by golden light. Imagine that you are sitting in a celestial field of light and space. Request the presence of the highest Self of the person whom you would like to forgive or ask forgiveness of. When their highest Self arrives, take a moment to center yourself by reconnecting with the gentle rise and fall of your abdomen. Allow yourself to offer a blessing, prayer, or forgiveness—or *ask* for forgiveness—in whatever way feels intuitive to you. Try not to force anything, let go of expectations. Trust the wisdom of your deeper Self to guide this communion and bring a force of healing. When you feel complete, ask the higher selves to return to their respective resting places. Begin to deepen your breath and slowly resurface from the meditation. Devote several minutes to freewriting afterward, followed by grounding with a cup of tea, walking barefoot on the earth, or a warm bath.

COMMUNITY PRACTICE: REMEMBERING ETHICS

It is said that samadhi (enlightenment) is not possible without the practice of the *yamas*.

The yamas are ethical principles that inspire and inform how we treat others. The Sanskrit word *yama* comes from the root word *yam*, which means "to hold back or turn away." These principles are so powerful that they are the foundation of the *niyamas*, which are principles for our relationship with ourselves. Our personal enlightenment is therefore dependent on how we care for and treat *all beings*. How we treat others extends to our thoughts, speech, and actions.

In a world where we are taught to look out "for number one," Western yoga practice itself has become tainted with individualism and disregard for the collective. But there is no yoga without the collective. The yamas are a full-spectrum practice; no part of our life should be separate from community care. The teachings tell us that we shouldn't act one way in the yoga studio, teaching a class, or with our spiritual friends (sangha) and then contradict our spiritual ethics when we are with our family, in a conflict, at work, or when none of our teachers or sangha is looking. Our ethical integrity, community care, and liberation are intrinsically tied together. This all becomes painfully obvious when harm is caused in yoga because of spiritual leaders forgetting, neglecting, or dismissing these concepts. Below you will find some suggestions of how to weave the practice of the yamas into family and communities.

Ahimsa (nonviolence) is the most important of the yamas. If you are not practicing nonviolence toward others, then the practice of all the other yamas and niyamas is futile. Ways of practicing nonviolence in the community can include being inclusive and honoring others' experiences and holding space for people to show up as their full selves, without judgment. Consider what actions may bring healing or spaciousness instead of increased friction when in conflict. Sharing your pronouns and land acknowledgments are helpful ways to model active ahimsa. Empower yourself to practice compassionate but firm boundaries to protect yourself and others.

Satya (truthfulness) in a community is speaking and communicating with clarity; not claiming to know things when you do not have complete information—knowing the difference between spreading rumors and sharing knowledge that may protect others from harm. Create space for people to share their voice, especially when it feels shaky or unsure. Practice being loving and compassionate in your truth-telling, which may mean you need to pause before speaking. Satya isn't about watering down your truth. It aligns with the energy of fierce compassion and allows that frequency to inform your words and delivery, especially when hard truth needs to be shared.

Asteya (nonstealing) is the practice of not taking, borrowing, or "tweaking" what doesn't belong to you. Stealing can take many forms. In a community, stealing can be as subtle as one person taking up the time of others in a self-indulgent way, leaving no time for others to share. Consistent and unapologetic lateness is also a form of stealing—you're wasting others' time. In the social media community, I have seen many examples of people giving lectures or workshops only to have their words paraphrased and turned into memes or reels and then shared without credit or the source cited. A beautiful antidote for asteya is to share your resources. Take a moment to acknowledge what resources, cultures, and people inspire you.

Brahmacharya (moderation of the senses and right use of energy) is often translated as "celibacy." Still, since most of us are probably not taking the vows of a renunciate—we're likely householders with the responsibilities of worldly life—when we consider the "right use of energy," the first inquiry is to highlight the many ways we experience distraction. Take a moment to consider the things that distract you—how do you waste time? *Note: Relaxing and resting is *not* a waste of time. It is a replenishing of energy, a reconnection to creativity and wholeness. Consider how you can be a source of presence, instead of a distraction, for your community. Are you the one who makes a joke to "lighten the mood" when a conversation gets serious and real? Or are you the one who has practiced how to drop in deeply to the divine spaciousness needed to process, feel, and integrate whatever is arising? How do you show up in community? Notice how some of your previous conditioning and samskaras show up in community spaces.

Aparigraha (nongreed) is the practice of not taking more than you need. Ask yourself, *How much do I need to be content, and what are my requirements for contentment based on?* Notice the emotions that arise when you feel that you do not have enough. Do you ever feel that you have too much? What do you consider to be your possessions in life? Are you considering your possessions to be other people—"my congregation," "my students"? Can you reframe the idea that you own land—"This is my land"—and instead embrace the concept that you are tending or stewarding the land as a living entity, not an inanimate object? This isn't about judging yourself for having abundance or feeling guilty for having more than others. Exploring the root of the desire to accumulate resources is an important step to cultivating a healthy relationship with the resources you have.

What actions can you take when you have too much of something? Practices that you may find helpful: join a community or neighborhood garden project where everyone shares the harvest; consider a seasonal purging of belongings and donations to charities; participate in clothes-swapping parties. When you genuinely don't have enough, empower yourself to ask for assistance. For deeper inquiry, ask yourself: What does it mean to possess inner abundance?

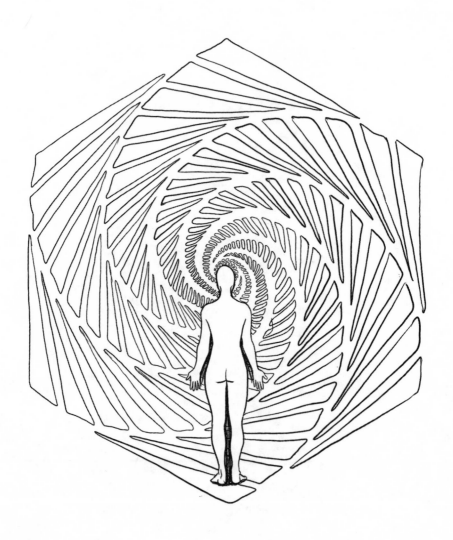

PART TWO

Portals and Practices

Am I asleep or am I awake?

Let me lean into the practices that fortify my
discernment

Remind me to turn my face toward the light of
divine intelligence.

The door to the prison cell is open

Attune me to the vibration of truth and amplify my
core frequency so I can taste my true nature

I trust that I can hold both fierce compassion and the power
to wield the sword to cut through any demon.

I lay down fear as I walk through the sacred portal
toward freedom.

I honor the transition

I reclaim my magic within the void

I only need to remember

Now, let me ask again

Am I asleep or am I awake?

MANY CULTURES HAVE RITUALS and ceremonies that require a pause in the normal activities of life to observe a transition from one life phase to the next. For example, many African cultures acknowledge birth, adulthood, marriage, eldership, and ancestorship with communal rituals. These ceremonies are rites of passage, marking the time that a person will be forever changed once the ceremony is complete, and the community holds them to the expectation of growth. When I think back to some transitional moments in my life—divorcing, embarking on a months-long spiritual journey to India, being fully present when my father took his last breath, accepting a new and sacred love into my life—these were all like walking through a portal to the unknown. They all began with a separation, whether forced or by conscious decision. I had to leave one way of existing in order to step into the unknown, while remaining open to stretching, growing, and learning. Consciously walking through transitional space is like being pulled apart and reassembled into a new form while being awake to every moment and allowing it to teach you. Most of the time in Western cultures when we experience unplanned life transitions, there are no rituals or ceremonies to hold us over the long periods of time needed to grow and heal. I suppose this is why I love yoga sadhana; it creates a spacious container for powerful insights, supporting us as we examine and integrate experiences of transformation. We may be given a prescription for a period of time to practice, such as forty to ninety days, but as the practices do their work, they also let us know when more time is needed, and we learn to deeply listen. Cultivating a relationship of honoring transitional space is a stepping-stone on the path toward spiritual maturity. The practices in this section of the book are all mini portals that can lead to greater awareness and understanding so that you can remember and reclaim your truest Self. Healing is not a linear journey, and neither is traveling through portals. There will be resistance and flow, forgetting and remembering, pain and joy. Allow these portals and practices to illuminate opportunities to grow and expand. As you move through these next chapters, remember to offer yourself grace. We are all coming from different life experiences, and it is possible that the contemplations and practices that may create space and insights may also bring up uncomfortable emotions. Remember to pause; check in with a trusted friend, mentor, or therapist if needed.

| 6 |

THE DO LIST

I AM FORTUNATE TO BE in sacred circles with hundreds of students for workshops and online retreats that I host either online or in person. We begin with an opening circle where I ask folks what they hope to receive and release during our time together. I like to create space for a responsive style of teaching, and even though I always have a planned theme of practice, I am also curious to understand what is most supportive for the collective. Every group has surprising collective commonalities and synchronicities. It's as if we were all called to the same place in time so that we could support one another in our healing. It has been essential for me, as a facilitator, to develop the skill of deep listening.

When teaching online and in-person retreats in 2022, I sensed a profound bone-deep exhaustion, despair, and anger about the state of the world and the fast pace of life that was making it hard to catch a breath. What I learned from students that year is that they had more than ever a deep longing to "connect to inner knowing and purpose." That longing was colored by the anxiety and self-doubt that can arise in a world that measures worthiness by performance, production, competition, comparison, and material success. As a culture, we can be obsessed with marking things off the to-do list that we believe will lead toward success and happiness. We need a reframe.

Maybe the practices we need most are the ones that awaken the remembrance of a place inside of us that is ancient, wise, whole, and eternally radiant. What if remembering that place was our purpose? Yoga practices can clear enough space so we can touch a tiny thread of our inner knowing and begin to intentionally and lovingly weave it through the whole of our life.

The longing to find purpose is a calling to remember your true Self. Yoga itself is remembrance, known in Sanskrit as *smarana*, "remembering the Divine within." We each have a seed of the universe in the cave of our heart. There is a difference between hoping this is true and remembering it. Some of the most powerful tools of remembrance are self-inquiry, yoga nidra, contemplation, and tantric practices. Several years ago, Charlie Morley—friend, lucid-dreaming teacher, and former Buddhist monk—shared a practice with me. I immediately recognized its deep power and clarity to support a practice of mind mapping that I had been doing for over a decade. Eventually it became a new *krama* (wise progression or succession) for my teaching. This practice, along with the mind-mapping practice I share in the next chapter, is the thread of remembrance that can infuse our life with meaning by inspiring us to live from the wisdom of the soul in every moment. It's a way to get clear on the most essential things to "do" for our soul and what to let go of.

DO AND DON'T DO PRACTICE

(5 minutes)

You can listen to this practice at www.shambhala.com/TheLuminousSelfPractices.
     To self-guide through the practice, set a timer for five minutes.
     Create two columns: "Do" on the left and "Don't Do" on the right.

Do	Don't Do

Start the timer and either close your eyes or soften your gaze. Bring your awareness inward and begin to notice your breath moving in and out of your body. Place one hand on your heart and your other hand on your belly. Let your attention rest on your abdomen. Notice how your navel rises and falls as your breath moves in and out. Feel your hand on your abdomen rising and falling. Feel all your breath moving in your belly as your chest becomes more and more still. (9 breaths)

This practice requires you to imagine that your life is ending. Take a few moments to recenter if needed and breathe deeply three times. If this brings up uncomfortable emotions, this is normal. If it feels like too much, please pause and come back to the exercise when and if you feel ready.

Imagine that you have learned that you have one year left to live. What would you do in that time? What would you immediately stop doing? Go to your chart and spend two minutes listing all of the things you would *do* and *stop doing* in that year.

Pause and stop writing ... Close your eyes and once again bring awareness to your heart. Breathe in and out three times from your heart center.

Imagine you have six months left. What would you do and not do? Write for ninety seconds.

Pause . . . Close your eyes and bring awareness to your heart. Breathe in and out three times from your heart center.

Imagine you have three months left. What would you do and not do? Write for one minute.

Pause . . . Close your eyes and bring awareness to your heart. Breathe in and out from your heart center in one breath.

Imagine you have one month left. What would you do and not do? Write for thirty seconds.

You have one week left. Write for fifteen seconds.

You have one day left. Write for ten seconds.

You have one minute left. Write for five seconds.

The practice is complete; please do not make any changes to what you have written.

INTENTIONAL PAUSE

Close your eyes or soften your gaze. Let your body receive nine deep belly breaths. Shake your body out for a few moments.

Take a moment to review your writing. What is the last word or phrase in the Do column? (1 minute left) Let's refer to this as your "Do Word."

SELF-INQUIRY

Take a few moments to write a short paragraph answering the following questions:

- Does this Do Word feel supportive and expansive, or does it feel contracting?
- If the Do Word feels contracting, is it representative of a pattern in life that you would like to shift? How can you begin to transform this pattern?

- How would your life change if you made your Do Word your *overarching* purpose, action, sentiment, or intention for everything you do from this day forward?
- Are you currently involved in a circumstance, whether it is a job, relationship, or project, that is *not* aligned with your Do Word?
- What needs to change in order for you to embrace this Do Word into your life?
- Where and how do you feel resistance to honoring the inner wisdom of your Do Word? Name the resistance. Is it a sensation, emotion, or feeling? Where did you feel resistance in your body as you moved through any part of the practice?
- What part of your life is currently most aligned with your Do Word?

We will be coming back to this Do Word soon. For now, set it aside and pause.

INTENTIONAL PAUSE: GROUNDING MOVEMENTS

Take a few minutes to ground yourself and allow the practice to integrate. You can do this by going outside and walking barefoot on the earth, dancing, or doing gentle yoga movements that bring you a sense of ease and steadiness.

THE PSYCHIC KNOTS

I was a bit freaked out when I was first introduced to the psychic knots, or *granthis* (pronounced "gruntis"). Somehow the idea of energetic knots that exist in my subtle body was a bit disconcerting. Because they exist in our energy body, if you cut your body open you will not find them, although sometimes people report feeling physical discomfort or sensations near the locations of the granthis. The word *granthi* can be translated to mean "doubt," "shackle," or "knot."[1] Psychic knots reside in the subtle body in four places, three of which are named after Hindu gods: Brahma, the creator; Vishnu, the preserver and sustainer; and Rudra, the one who eradicates problems from their roots. These knots are made up of the same samskaras, vasanas, and karmas we explored in chapter 2. The knots are similar to stuck, entangled, deep-seated balls of energy that restrict the free flow of energy and freedom in our subtle body (nadis, chakras, and vayus), which prevents *kundalini shakti*— the awakening force of consciousness that burns through our limitations— from rising. This affects us at every level of our being and consciousness. To transcend our conditioning, we should recognize the existence of these knots and begin the work of cutting them free. Some of the resistance we feel in moving toward the power and wisdom of true Self is because these knots have created blockages in our psychic and subtle energy. Our higher Self becomes obscured from our view when we are stuck in the illusion of personality, ego, likes and dislikes, greed, and aversion. Granthis are the energetic and psychic manifestations of avidya (misperception). When any of these granthis are pierced or cut, we begin to expand our consciousness and recognize our true nature. We can slowly become free of our energetic blockages and begin to experience life with more awareness.

Brahma granthi is located at the base of the spine at the root chakra (*muladhara*), and it can manifest as an attachment to worldly things, materialism, fear of death, and lack of basic needs being met. This granthi creates anxiety, instability, fight-or-flight response, and a sense of groundlessness.

Vishnu granthi is located between the navel and the throat center, encompassing the navel, heart, and throat chakras. This granthi can manifest as the accumulation of personal power and possessions; hoarding of wealth; and attachment to people, ego, control, and status. When we experience the effects of this granthi, we focus more on outer purpose than inner purpose. We remain focused on individuality, self-centeredness, and power.

Rudra granthi is located at the third-eye point. It relates to pride in intellect, knowledge, or service to others. With this granthi, we experience the world as dualistic, and we lack the vision for unity and equality. We may become attached to psychic visions or our intellect. We can be transactional in our acts of service because they are not rooted in karma yoga. We like to accumulate knowledge but do not have the clarity of self-knowledge. This leaves us bound to our biases, opinions, and martyrdom.

Hridaya granthi is located at the spiritual heart center; it is not the same as Vishnu granthi or the physical location of the heart organ. The spiritual heart center is also the place of *hridaya guha*, the cave of the heart where the microcosm of the entire universe exists.[2] There, we can experience direct knowledge and remembrance of the true Self. Hridaya is where the Self or Atman is remembered. The Chandogya Upanishad says, "This Atman is smaller than a grain of paddy, than a barley corn, a mustard seed. . . . This Atman residing in the heart is greater than the earth, greater than the sky, greater than heaven, greater than all of these worlds."[3] When this knot is tied up, we believe *I am the body* or *This is mine*, and we are caught in the web of avidya.[4] When this is dissolved, we realize the true Self.

> Releasing the knots of the heart is also the dissolution of the subtle body and going beyond all karma.
>
> —*Vamadeva David Frawley*[5]

HOW DO THESE KNOTS RELATE TO OUR PURPOSE?

When we feel "stuck," our creativity, inspiration, stability, and ability to love unconditionally can feel muted. We are separated from the muse of our heart. We have a hard time realizing our true potential when these knots are all tied up. Quite simply, our consciousness is blocked from expanding while these knots are still in place. Some teachings say that these knots are in place to keep the kundalini energy from rising too fast, but we can begin to untie these knots with gentle practices that are spoken about in the tantric texts, specifically the *Hatha Yoga Pradipika*. I recommend exploring these practices gently and practicing self-inquiry after each one. Understand that these practices can release many emotional, mental, and subtle energies; slow is the way to go.

SELF-INQUIRY

Here are a few questions to get you started:

- What are you noticing about each of the centers where the knots reside prior to practice? Do they feel constricted, open, disregarded?
- How often are you aware of these centers in your body?
- What do you notice after practice? Is there a release of emotion, pain, or memories? Devote a few minutes of freewriting after each practice to help integrate your experiences.

BHASTRIKA PRANAYAMA

This kumbhaka called bhastrika enables the three granthis (psychic/pranic knots) to be broken.

—*Hatha Yoga Pradipika 2:67*[6]

Bhastrika is known as "bellows breath." Before practicing, take a moment to close your eyes and imagine a bellow used to stoke a fire. See the action of the bellows chamber filling with air and expelling air as you pump the handles. The intake and release of air are forceful yet equal, unlike other breaths like *Kapalabhati* (skull-shining breath, or breath of fire), where only the exhale is forceful.

- Find a comfortable meditation shape and allow your spine to be tall and supported by a chair or wall if necessary. Place your hands on your belly and take a few moments to notice your natural breath. Feel your belly

naturally rising and falling as you breathe in and out. Invite stillness into the body.
- Begin to intentionally expand your belly fully as you inhale.
- Exhale forcefully through your nose, releasing all the air.
- With the same force, inhale, expanding your belly.
- Continue to forcefully inhale and exhale equally for ten rounds. You may notice a slight hissing sound.
- End with one slow deep breath in and out.

Benefits: Strengthens the nervous system; harmonizes emotions; establishes witness consciousness, clarity of mind, and physical vitality.[7]

Note: This practice is contraindicated for those who are pregnant or have high blood pressure. This practice can also feel similar to hyperventilation. Be cautious if you experience panic attacks or anxiety.

BANDHAS

Bandhas are energy locks done with the physical body to help redirect the flow of vital life force to specific places in the body. Three primary bandhas are performed at the base of the spine, abdomen, and throat—correlating to the location of the three granthis. These help unlock the energy and knots at the granthis. When they are performed together, they are known as Maha Mudra, the Great Symbol or Gesture. These bandhas are best learned with a skilled teacher. You will find resources in the back of the book for video links.

JALANDHARA BANDHA (THROAT LOCK)

- Find a comfortable meditation shape and allow your spine to be tall and supported by a chair or wall if necessary. Spend a few moments to notice your natural breath.
- Let your hands rest on your knees, palms facing down.

- Continue to notice your breath moving in and out and allow your sternum to lift as you inhale.
- On your next inhale, about two-thirds of your lung capacity, hold your breath at the top of the inhale and lower your chin to your chest. Press your palms into your knees as you draw your chin in and back; the back of your neck stays long. Slightly round your shoulders forward to deepen the lock.
- When you need to, release and exhale.
- Practice the throat lock twice more.

Benefits: Improves concentration and clarity and increases breath retention.

Note: This practice is contraindicated for any injury to the neck, vertigo, cardiac issues, or high blood pressure.

UDDIYANA BANDHA (ABDOMINAL LOCK)

- Find a comfortable meditation shape.
- Allow your hands to rest gently on your knees. If you are standing, widen your stance to just beyond hip distance, bend your knees, keep your spine long, and rest your hands on your knees.
- Inhale through your nose and exhale through your mouth a few times.
- Inhale through your nose and exhale through your mouth with a *whoosh* sound. Feel as though you are emptying both your stomach and your lungs of all air as you suspend your breath out.
- Resist the urge to inhale. Suspending your breath out, begin to draw your navel in and up. Feel your navel drawing back toward your spine and up. Your upper abdomen will become concave and hollow.
- Slowly release your belly before the next inhale to avoid gasping.

Benefits: Strengthens willpower; purifies toxins in the abdomen; aids digestion and mental and physical assimilation.

Note: This practice is contraindicated for pregnancy, ulcers, irritable bowel syndrome (IBS), and high blood pressure.

MULA BANDHA (ROOT LOCK)

- Find a comfortable meditation shape on a chair or in your favorite seated posture.
- As you inhale, begin to contract and lift the muscles of your pelvic floor by engaging your perineal muscles. As you exhale, release your perineal muscles.
- Practice engaging and releasing your perineum as you inhale and exhale. Inhale, engage. Exhale, release.
- While breathing in slowly, draw your pelvic floor muscles up, contracting your perineum for three counts.

Benefits: Stabilizes and calms.

Note: This practice is contraindicated for pregnancy, high blood pressure, abdominal issues, and possibly menstruation.

INTENTIONAL PAUSE: SELF-INQUIRY

Take a moment to review your Do Word. Which knots do you intuitively feel may be related to this Do Word? How and why? This may be the one to focus on first. Take some time to explore the related practices before moving on to the next chapter, where we will learn the ritual of weaving this thread of the Do Word throughout everything in your life. The next chapter will explore how to integrate your Do Word into your community care.

| 7 |

THE AUSPICIOUS MIND MAP

I WAS INTRODUCED TO THE PRACTICE of mind mapping by my dear friend Isabelle over twenty years ago. I have been using mind maps over the years, and daily for the last several, because I have found the practice to be a powerful ritual for weaving my truth through everything I do and birthing ideas, projects, and dreams to fruition. The term *mind mapping*, first coined by the psychologist Tony Buzan in 1974, is also known as radiant thinking. Mind mapping is usually considered a visual thinking tool and a way to organize the relationship of ideas around a central concept. Similar methods were used by Leonardo da Vinci and Albert Einstein. When centered around a concept that is authentic to the core of your being, it is a powerful way to stay aligned with your truth and infuse everything you do with the fragrance of divine action.

In mind mapping, one central idea, word, or concept blossoms into other thoughts, inspirations, and concepts. Your central word will be your Do Word as the frequency that informs everything else. You can think of it as the underlying note that plays beneath everything you do. How does a mind map become more than just a brainstorming tool? How does it actually move us toward an auspicious life? When we make our Do Word the central

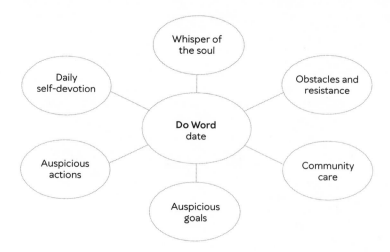

focus of our mind map, the mind map becomes a ritual that adds depth and meaning in our daily life. It serves as a reminder that whatever is most important in our lives should weave through and inform our lives and actions in meaningful ways. Your Do Word will be the central concept that radiates out to six other auspicious categories that can help you remain centered, amplify discernment, create healthy boundaries, and sustainably move toward your goals and dreams.

THE SIX AUSPICIOUS CATEGORIES

There are six auspicious categories to begin to your mind map journey.[1] After you have spent some time working with these six categories, you may be inspired to add to them, but for the first mind map sadhana please explore and become familiar with the categories suggested below.

1. Whisper of the Soul

When was the last time you had a profound inspiration or a flash of intuition that felt like a deep inner knowing? What were you doing when it happened?

You may have been intensely focused on one thing or on nothing at all. There is no telling how a whisper of the soul drops into our awareness from "out of nowhere." Was it there all along or did we just get quiet, still, and spacious enough to hear, feel, or sense it? When has wisdom dropped in for you in the past? You may have been meditating, practicing yoga asana, dancing, walking in nature, running, chanting, dreaming, or hiking. Sitting with the contemplations below may help you remember when and how you may have received whispers of the soul in the past.

INTENTIONAL PAUSE: SOUL WHISPER CONTEMPLATION

- Recall three times in the past ten to twenty years when you felt you had a whisper from the soul, an inner knowing or epiphany. How did it come to you? Was the information you received audible, visual, or sensory?
- Take a moment to write down three whispers you received from the soul and approximately when they occurred. What were you doing when you received them? Why were they so profound? How did/does this wisdom help to guide you?

When you have a better sense of how you might connect to your whispers of the soul, you can commit to a daily meditation or other practice that allows you to create an inner opening. I also recommend the Soul Whisper Meditation on page 163, which is also available in audio here: www.shambhala.com/TheLuminousSelfPractices.

2. Daily Self-Devotion—The Doorway to Expansion

Choose one thing that you can do daily to honor and love yourself. A simple act of daily self-devotion is a reminder that you are deserving of daily tending. Self-devotion is counter-culture and can help us feel more resourced to nourish ourselves. How you choose to practice self-devotion is personal and should be anchored and aligned with your Do Word.

My Do Word is *love*, so when I consider how I want to practice self-devotion, it is always infused with love. I may offer gratitude for the many ways I experience love in my life. I may use an affirmation that reminds me that I am love. My self-devotion is a daily practice; it could be five minutes or an hour. Doing a self-devotion practice daily is key; it will amplify your feelings of worthiness and help you to create sacred boundaries. Examples are warm-oil self-massage, walks in nature, dancing or movement, preparing a nourishing meal, a ritual bath, or resting—anything that is inspiring and healing for you!

3. Auspicious Goals

Auspicious goals are the dreams, goals, and visions you have for the future. They can be very specific—"I will complete my book proposal by X date," "I have a nurturing home that is supportive and healing and well within my financial means," or even as simple as "I am in radiant health." I suggest starting with just one auspicious goal for the first three days of practice. The goal will stay the same. Every day you'll create a new mind map. Remember, it's a daily ritual.

Your Do Word informs how you approach moving toward your auspicious goal. Notice as you integrate the mind map into your daily life that the "goal" may refine itself. You may become aware of how your goal may need to shift slightly to become better aligned with your Do Word. It's not uncommon that we may realize that our goals keep us stuck in unhelpful patterns. Let go of the desire to try to extract as much as possible from your practice as quickly as possible. Be patient. We have a manifestation obsession in wellness culture and are constantly trying to " manifest" without an understanding of the true desire beneath, and that can create problems. Is your auspicious goal in alignment with the whispers of your soul, or is it what dominant culture tells you will make you valuable and relevant? Let go of any feeling that you want to "get something" and instead connect to your Do Word and let that soften your grasping or sense of urgency. You will find the energy of extraction to ultimately be contracting rather than expansive. As you consider your auspicious goal, check in with yourself and notice if you are being motivated by what others think you "should" be doing, competing with others, or creating goals that are informed by old stories and pain. When we are unaware of our samskaras and vasanas that create the small self, we can unconsciously recreate similar patterns that caused us discomfort in the past. Take time to notice what happens in your body when you consider your auspicious goals. What does it *feel* like in your body—expansive, freeing, joyful, or suffocating?

4. Obstacles and Resistance

It is natural to have obstacles and feel resistance to growth. But it is not often that we shine a light on our resistances as a daily practice. I find that naming my obstacles and inner resistance helps to diminish their power over me. Acknowledging the obstacles and resistances we face allows us to begin to identify patterns and skillfully create antidotes to whatever is getting in our way. Once we identify obstacles, we can integrate helpful practices to overcome them or lessen their impact on our life.

It is important to acknowledge the overarching obstacles that affect culture at large. It is also crucial to drill down on our personal resistances that are here as daily teachers on our path. Those can look like procrastination, disorganization, forgetfulness, carelessness, untended grief, distraction, or lack of resources. Sometimes our obstacles have been with us for so long that it seems they may never change. But once we bring awareness to them, without shame or judgment, we can begin to see that they are not static. There is a pulsation in every energy, including resistance, that allows us to shift our relationship to it and to find ways to work within it. Naming our obstacles can help us move beyond the spiritual bypassing that can happen when we get deep into our spiritual work and it starts to feel sticky. When we encounter resistance, we have choices: we can turn away, light some incense, and hope for the best; we can try to force our way through it; or we can pause and find an antidote that will help us dissolve the resistance, which may include asking for help.

5. Auspicious Actions—Creating Momentum toward Freedom

Auspicious actions are the intentional actions you take to provide antidotes to your daily resistance and obstacles as well as to help you move toward auspicious goals and follow the whispers of the soul. Auspicious actions are the most important part of the mind map and should always align with the center circle—your Do Word.

Auspicious actions are not a traditional to-do list. They are actions that bring presence to each day to help you to grow in a positive direction and remain in alignment with your Do Word. They help you to release stagnancy, forgetfulness, and doubt. Auspicious actions need not be grand actions; think of them more like micro actions that over time will accumulate into momentum. You must have at least one action to help ease the obstacles and resistance you may be facing.

SELF-INQUIRY

Take some time to consider the following questions to help you complete your auspicious actions circle:

- What action would best serve the whispers of the soul?
- What actions or antidotes would help to ease the resistance you are experiencing from obstacles?
- What is one thing you can do today to honor your auspicious goal?
- How can you approach these actions with the quality of your Do Word?

FINDING THE ANTIDOTE CONTEMPLATIONS

Below I've listed a few common ways resistance shows up and actions we can explore to help dissolve it. You many notice that some of these common resistances are callbacks to sutra 1:30 and the nine obstacles (page 46) that are impediments to transformation.

Type of Resistance: Procrastination | Auspicious Action: Movement

List the ways you procrastinate and distract yourself. Commit to leaving one of those behind and using the time to move your physical body in some way—dancing, walking, yoga, swimming. If you are unable to move your body, consider receiving a massage or physical therapy. Once you are done with movement, spend a few minutes doing something that you have been putting off. Start small. If you have a huge organization or cleaning project, for example, pick one thing from the pile and file it or throw it away. If you find yourself procrastinating because of indecision or restlessness, speak with a wise friend or mentor who may be able to help you focus and make choices.

Type of Resistance: Doubt | Auspicious Action: Anything That Helps You Gain Clarity

What does it feel like in your body and mind when you experience clarity of thought? Take a moment to remember the times in your life that you had the most clarity. What were the circumstances? How did this affect your life? Was there ever a time when you felt very sure of a direction that you wanted to move in and someone convinced you otherwise? It's important to understand what "clears your mind." Try five to ten minutes of daily morning meditation followed by freewriting. Dance or shake for five minutes. Connect with your wise friends, elders in your community, or a trusted therapist to air out confusion and cyclical thinking. Make a list of what it is that you have absolute faith in. How can any of this faith list be helpful in overcoming doubt? Contemplate where your doubt stems from.

Type of Resistance: Fear | Auspicious Action: Summoning Courage

First, name your fear. Devote a few moments to writing about what you are afraid of. Then pause for a moment, drawing your awareness inward, and remember the last time you felt courage or strength, whether physical, mental, or spiritual. Remember what it was that you were doing at the time. Now just tap into the feeling. Let the circumstances go; just be with the feeling for one minute. Notice how courage, power, and strength are still alive within you.

SELF-INQUIRY

What is one thing that you have the courage to do today? This doesn't have to be a big action. Remember yourself as courageous and strong and imagine how you could move through fear. Devote a few minutes to writing a short story (just a paragraph or two) of how you imagine moving through fear. When you are finished, circle a few of the active words. Notice if you can embrace any of these words as auspicious actions and antidotes to add to your mind map.

Type of Resistance: Anger | Auspicious Action: Cultivating Compassion

Sometimes the compassion we need to cultivate is first for ourselves. Take a moment to consider all of the ways that you deny yourself compassion.

When do you feel others are deserving of your compassion, and how do you withhold compassion? Is your anger tied to an event of the past or the present moment? Journal about your anger and how past grievances may be coloring your life. Offer yourself grace. Anger is a human emotion that needs to be held in divine acceptance before we can shift it. Practice tonglen or spend time serving those in need. Read Lama Rod Owen's book *Love and Rage*.

Type of Resistance: Urgency | Auspicious Action: Cultivating Patience and Spaciousness

Unanswered urgency is often met with shame, disappointment, judgment, fear of failure, and fear of missing out. On our spiritual journey, we transform the sense of urgency with space, acceptance, and the understanding that the path to healing is not linear. Take your time to pause and reflect often. Practice meditation, yoga nidra, and silence. Let go of intractable timelines, manage expectations, and create sacred boundaries. Get to know your internal cycles and seasons; we all have times of natural ebbs and flow during each day, season, and year. Learn to honor and deeply listen to the wisdom of your body and the season of your life. Take sabbaticals from answering emails or social media. Read Octavia Raheem's book *Pause, Rest, Be*.

6. Community Care

The circle of community care is a way for you to share the essence of your Do Word with your community. The best way to begin is to ask yourself, *What does my community need? How can they be nourished by my Do Word?* This can be as simple as a prayer, a compassionate gesture, volunteering, donating, or practicing the Connected Roots Meditation (p. 61). You can offer the fruits of your practice to your community after meditation, symbolically, by remembering this prayer at the end of each meditation or yoga practice: *May the fruits of my practice be surrendered for the liberation of all beings.* Create opportunities for friends and family to gather. Community care is soul care. When we remember our soul, we remember the soul of the universe.

THE RITUAL OF MIND MAPPING

Daily rituals support transformation. Ritual can hold you in times of uncertainty. The practice of mind mapping or any practice done with consistency and reverence becomes a ritual that opens the portal to deeper levels of awareness. The power of the auspicious mind map is that it is centered around your last desire in your (imagined) moment of death—a moment where you know that there is nothing more you can take from life. What you choose to do in that moment says a lot about how you wish to live while you still can.

We can be so distracted by the doings of life that we forget our call to live a life of meaning. Not only is the mind map a tool of remembrance of that imagined moment of death but it also centers the truth that tomorrow is not promised. It propels us to live into our truth with everything we do. This is a daily *tapasya*—a practice that generates the heat of transformation. It can bring up a lot of resistance—and change. I recommend doing this practice of mind mapping for a period of forty to ninety consecutive days to begin. Notice what changes. If you notice significant change, continue with it. Science suggests that neural pathways in the brain take forty to seventy days to change and create new habits.[2] Again, we in the West are usually not accustomed to doing things with consistency over long periods of time with devotion. So if you are feeling resistance, this is the first point of inquiry for you. Why? The practice will take about five to ten minutes a day. There is no wrong way to proceed. If you miss a day, keep going! If you aren't sure that you can make it for forty days, commit to seven days to begin or ask a friend to join you. It is the daily dedication to your Do Word that reveals a continuum of healing that is connected to the web of life.

As much as the body requires food for nourishment, our souls and spirits require ritual to stay whole.

—*Malidoma Patrice Somé*[3]

| 8 |

EMBRACING TRANSITION

Yoga is the practice of preparing to die gracefully.
—*Gary Kraftsow*[1]

LIFE IS TRANSITION. The word *transition* derives from the fifteenth-century Latin for "to go across" or "to go over." There are so many transitions in life that they can be easy to miss because we haven't learned to honor them. Many times we may be aware of a transition point in life because it feels like a crossroads—a moment in life when we become acutely aware that things can't stay the same. This crossroads *demands* that we pause. But the pace of life tells us that we cannot pause; we need to get on with it and hurry up. Pausing creates the spaciousness for reflection, acceptance, and visioning. And while we stand in the murkiness of the unknown, it might feel like part of us is being pulled apart or dying. Remembering asks us to be present to the fact that we are ever closer to death and inspires us to live in a more meaningful way.

The most significant transition that we will ever experience is death. Let's get that right out there—death cannot be avoided. As much as we might like to pretend that we will live forever, our time in this physical body is limited. Contemplating this fact is not morbid; it is an opportunity to commit to being more awake, heart-centered, and intentional in this life. When we deny the reality of the impermanence of life, we suffer.

Indigenous cultures have much to teach us about our relationship with death. They remind us that honoring the cycles of nature and practicing rituals of grieving when our loved ones or members of our community pass on is a vital part of life that we in the West have mostly forgotten. In the Dagara tribe of West Africa, it is considered criminal to go on with "business as usual" when a person dies.[2] The grieving rituals last for days and include the entire village. In the Jewish culture, when someone dies, it is customary to "sit shiva"; *shiva* means "seven" and refers to a ritual of seven days of mourning. It is a time for those who have lost loved ones to heal, receive condolences, and be supported by the community. When a dear one dies, it is a time for us to remember our loved ones and pray for them, and this inevitably leads us to contemplate our own death and the meaning of our life.

There is power in pausing to observe, honor, and soften into the transitions between what we know and what has not yet become. If we can intentionally cultivate a relationship with this liminal space, we may open portals to new awareness. There is always a part of us that is dying and another part that is waiting to be born.

> Each moment arises directly from infinity
> Each moment dissolves directly into infinity
> The next moment also arises directly from infinity
> Concentration on what is between the dissolution of the prior
>   moment and the arising of the subsequent moment opens the
>   gateway to infinity.
>
> —*Swami Veda Bharati*[3]

INTENTIONAL PAUSE

The contemplation of death brings the question of *Who am I?* front and center: *What part of me dies, and what part of me will remain? What part of me is witnessing the dying? Can I connect to the eternal part of me while I am still in this body?*

We experience little deaths, voids, and transitions daily that we don't even realize. When we learn to observe these gaps, it awakens us to life. One of the most recurrent and sometimes less obvious voids is the space between the breaths. Each breath offers us an opportunity to observe the pause between the exhale and inhale and to rest and surrender into the space of the unknown for just a moment. Each exhale released out is a form of dying, a completion of a cycle. Each inhale received is a rebirth, renewal, and a beginning of a new cycle. The space between can be our greatest teacher. The breath cycle mimics nature—the sun rising and setting, the moon rising and setting, a whole day beginning and coming to completion. The stars in our universe are constantly dying and being born. Some of the stars we see in the night sky have already died, their light extinguished, but we are still receiving the frequencies of light because they are so many light years away. Galaxies are born and die over millennia. If you observe nature, there are no hard stops or starts to the transitions of death or birth. Things go fallow; there is a progression to life, an unfolding of beauty that we must learn to become awake to in every moment. There is a part of you that remembers what it feels like to die and a part of you that remembers what it feels like to be born. Each ritual or practice we devote ourselves to allows us to observe the slow progression of releasing, letting go, composting what is dying, and welcoming what wants to be born. When we are awake to these cycles, we can be purposeful about the seeds we are planting and the energy we give to what is trying to emerge. We can practice accepting what is falling away and have clarity about how clinging can deplete our life force. We can also stop watering the seeds that are harmful to us and others.

The observation of dying and death in practice can be overwhelming, so let's start with practices to gently shift our awareness of what it means to embrace and observe transition. We can begin with the one gift we all have access to—the breath.

SPACE BETWEEN BREATH PRACTICE

(approx. 10–15 minutes)

You can find audio of this practice at www.shambhala.com/TheLuminousSelf Practices.

Find a comfortable, accessible seat, or lie down on your back in a comfortable position.

Begin to observe your body breathing; this means letting go of the "doing" of breathing.

Reframe your intention from *taking* a breath to *receiving* a breath. *Let the breath come to you.* There is nothing you need to do to earn it. As you release your breath on exhale, feel yourself giving back to the natural world around you. Notice a softening within you. Notice the quality of your mind as you soften to allow yourself to receive and release your breath in this way.

Observe yourself receiving and releasing breath while noticing the gentle rise and fall of your navel. Feel your navel rising and falling effortlessly. (10 breaths)

Now begin to notice the direction of your breath. Notice how the inhale descends, and the exhale ascends. You don't need to do anything to make this happen or to try to shape your breath. Just notice the movement of your breath within your body. (10 breaths)

Begin to observe the flow of your breath. Feel the tip of your nose and follow the flow of your breath from the moment it enters your nostrils, rides along the roof of your nose, fills your lungs, and then dissolves.

Notice the natural impulse to release your breath. Follow that flow of your breath as it reaches your nose and exits your nostrils. Notice how your breath moves outside your body and eventually dissolves. (10 breaths)

Now let your attention rest on the space between the breaths. Feel as though you can rest in the space between the inhale and exhale. And the space between the exhale and inhale. You are not doing any kind of retention or suspension of your breath. As you become aware of the space between the breaths, you are softening, surrendering into that void space. All of your attention is now inside of the transitions between the breaths, not the breath flow. Rest and soften in the space between. (10 breaths)

Now continue to observe your breath and the space between; allow yourself to observe the arrival or departure of the next breath and the transitions as they come and go. Feel the place where the in-breath arrives. Maybe you sense the in-breath arriving from a point outside of the body (not right at the opening of your nostrils). Notice how far the out-breath travels as you receive and release, feeling it travel to back to an infinite space. (10 breaths)

Begin to notice the whole of your body from the tip of your toes to the top of your head and back down to your toes. Begin to feel your entire body filling with breath. When you are ready, come back to sitting.

INTENTIONAL PAUSE: SELF-INQUIRY

Devote a few minutes to freewriting about your experience:

- What part of your breath did you find most challenging—receiving or releasing the breath?
- Does this challenge in either receiving or releasing mirror itself in your daily life? Are you comfortable receiving from others? Are your closest friendships transactional or unconditional? Are you able to release judgment, grudges, and resentments easily? Is it easier for you to give than to receive? How did it feel to pause between the breaths? Where and how did you experience freedom or constriction?
- Do you have more tension in daily life when things are beginning or ending?

- What did you learn from "the space between"?
- Did your mind become still or more agitated in the space between the breaths?
- What part of you is dying, and what part of you is waiting to be born?

As you move on to the next practices, please take time to explore each practice. Don't try to do them all in the same day. Over the next week or so, practice one of these each day, devote ample time to freewriting and self-inquiry, and see which practices resonate with you most.

THE DEATH OF THOUGHT AND THE NON-SELF

Sometimes it is helpful to actively negate thoughts as they arise to create an intentional void. In that void space, free of thoughts and distraction, we may be able to glimpse the light of truth. We have already explored this with the practices of cultivating the opposite and creating antidotes to our resistances. When we negate everything that is not Divine Consciousness, we eventually land in a place that is nondual, dissolving the illusion of separateness from the universe, nature, and the true Self. Similar to the Who Am I Not? Practice in chapter 2 (page 22), finding the truth about the nature of the inner Self is a path to negating all the thoughts about it, as the true Self cannot be described. The practice of *neti neti*, which translates to "not this, not that (this)," is a powerful jnana yoga (the yoga of knowledge) practice that is referred to in the Upanishads and *Avadhuta Gita*. This practice is considered a search that reduces the possibilities of what constitutes truth through the process of elimination. As we continue to negate the thoughts, feelings, images, bodily sensations, and elemental qualities, we realize that the truth of the Divine is not this and not that. Ascribing qualities to the divine Self is beyond our capacity.

Atman is "neither this, nor this" (neti, neti). The Self cannot be described in any way. Na-it—that is neti. It is through this process of neti, neti that you give up everything—the cosmos, the body, the mind, and everything—to realize the Self.
—*Brihadaranyaka Upanishad*[4]

tattvamasyādi-vākyena svātmā hi pratipāditaḥ, neti neti śrutir-brūyāt-anṛtaṁ pāñca-bhautikam.

The saying, "That thou art" asserts the reality of your true Self. The saying, "not this, not this" negates the reality of the five elements.
—*Avadhuta Gita 1:25*[5]

NETI NETI PRACTICE

(approx. 15–20 minutes)

You can find audio of this practice at www.shambhala.com/TheLuminousSelf Practices.

Begin the practice by finding a comfortable meditation posture where you can remain alert and stable. Devote a few moments to observing your breath. Let go of judgment or trying to shape your breath in any way. Allow your breath to flow in and out effortlessly. Observe the rise and fall of the navel on the inhale and exhale. (2 minutes)

Begin to invite stillness into your body with each inhale and exhale. Even though your outer body may move or adjust, begin to feel an inner calm unfolding.

Bring your awareness to your physical body and scan your body from your toes to the top of your head and back to your toes. When any distraction arises in your awareness—a sound, image, thought, or anything—repeat "Neti neti" silently to yourself while remembering the meaning, "Not this, not that," and releasing the distraction. (1 minute)

Bring your awareness to the space outside of your body. Anytime you notice anything come into your awareness—a sound, image, or thought—repeat "Neti neti" silently while remembering the meaning, "Not this, not that." (1 minute)

Rest your attention at your heart center. Anytime that anything comes into your awareness—a sound, image, or thought—repeat "Neti, neti" silently to yourself while remembering the meaning, "Not this, not that." (3 minutes)

Lastly, continue neti neti without focusing awareness on any particular place. (3 minutes)

Slowly come back by receiving and releasing a few deep breaths, then devoting a few minutes to freewriting.

INTENTIONAL PAUSE: SELF-INQUIRY

Consider the following questions:

- Were there any recurring thoughts or feelings that you noticed?
- What surprised you most about your experience in the practice?
- Did you experience any resistance during this practice? If so, when and how?

FINDING THE INNER SILENCE

The fifth limb of yoga is known as pratyahara, or withdrawal of the senses. As the fifth limb, pratyahara is the bridge that allows us to cross from the physical external practices of yoga over to the deeper, inner stages of yoga—one-pointed focus (*dharana*), meditation (*dhyana*), and the final goal of samadhi (enlightenment or liberation).[6] Pratyahara creates a natural transition or void space between the two and is a powerful practice because the mind and the senses are connected. If we withdraw our senses inward, we limit our mind's ability to experience the outside world, and instead, our mind begins to turn toward our inner landscape. Our mind can become aware of its original calm and luminous nature.

There are three types of pratyahara—physical, mental, and pranic. We can think of them as stages or distinct kinds of practices. We can withdraw our attention from our physical senses and establish witness consciousness in physical pratyahara. We practice mental pratyahara by withdrawing our mental awareness away from our thoughts (e.g., neti neti). Or we can withdraw energy from an object such as our physical body (e.g., yoga nidra) for pranic pratyahara.

In my practice, the practices of inner silence, specifically *antar mouna* (inner silence), were game changers. One of my first teachers introduced me to antar mouna over twenty years ago. I then explored the practice again during the pandemic with one of my teachers, Swami Premajyoti Saraswati. It is a beautiful practice to experience pratyahara and cultivate a peaceful mind. The following practice is a simplified version of antar mouna. The practice guides us into observing the mind and learning how we can witness our senses instead of being drawn toward them and brought out into the external world of distraction.

INNER SILENCE PRACTICE
(approx. 15–20 minutes)

You can find audio of this practice at www.shambhala.com/TheLuminousSelf Practices.

Find your comfortable seat, leaning against a wall or sitting in a chair to support your back. You can also try this lying down if sitting isn't comfortable. As you find comfort, allow your awareness to move toward your breath. Feel and sense that your body is breathing effortlessly. Bring your attention to the opening of your nostrils. Feel the moment the air touches your nostrils. As you feel your body exhale, feel the moment that your breath leaves your nostrils. Keep your awareness at the opening of your nostrils. Feel the touch of breath, the air, as it moves in and out. (3 breaths)

Now, shift attention to your left nostril with the power of your mind or your imagination—awareness at your left nostril. Feel as though you can breathe in through your left nostril and out through your right. Inhale through your right. Exhale through your left. Inhale left, exhale right. Inhale right, exhale left. Inhale left, exhale right. Inhale right, exhale left.

Now allow the breath to flow through both nostrils. Feel the natural flow of breath moving in and out of both nostrils. Feel your body soften just a little. Forehead softens, shoulders, jaw. Continue to notice your breath moving in and out through both nostrils.

Feel your body become very, very heavy, almost as though your body is as steady as a rock. If this makes you uncomfortable in any way, let it go and continue to observe your breath.

Begin to feel the sensation of cloth, of your clothing, touching your skin. Feel a point on your body where the fabric touches your skin. Feel as though you are receiving that touch of the cloth on your skin. Then release that feeling of the cloth on your skin and move to another point on your body where you feel the cloth touching your skin. Feel as though you are receiving this touch, this feeling of the cloth on your skin, and then release that feeling of touch and move to another point where you feel the cloth touching your skin. Continue in this way. (2 minutes)

Allow your attention to move to outside sounds. Hear all the sounds outside the room that you are sitting in. Land on any sound. Notice the sound. Now be aware of what the sound is and feel as though you are receiving the sound. Release the sound and move your awareness to another sound. Landing on a new sound, acknowledge what the sound is. Feel as though you are receiving the sound, and then release the sound. Continue allowing your awareness to move from sound to sound in this way: landing, acknowledging what the sound is, receiving, and then letting it go. (2 minutes)

Continue to sit quietly and allow spontaneous thoughts to flow. Without getting involved in the story of the thoughts, notice the thoughts as they arise and allow them to release. You are observing the flow of the thoughts as a witness.

Gently move your awareness to the space of *chidakasha* (the space of consciousness), which is the space just behind your forehead. Imagine that your forehead is this blank, dark screen. Gaze into the space behind your forehead, sensing that space, dark like the night sky. You are the observer, gazing into the space of the night sky behind your forehead. Be aware of any images or colors, feelings, or sensations. Be the observer. Don't let these images, feelings, or thoughts carry you away. Receive and release. Stay in the space of the observer as you gaze into the dark space of the night sky behind your forehead. (2 minutes)

Now slowly just begin to come back. Deepening your breath with full-body awareness, feeling as though you can bring self-awareness back to your body from the tip of your toes to the top of your head. And as you come back to that full-body awareness, chant the mantra OM. (3 times)

Take a deep breath.

Chant OM. (3 times)

Take as much time as you need to come back gently, and please take the next three minutes or so to freewrite.

INTENTIONAL PAUSE

Take some time to move your body or take a walk outside before continuing to the next section. Let the prior practice fully integrate and land in your nervous system. See if you can devote ten minutes to releasing the need to use any devices, check emails, or converse with others. Be with the silence.

DEATH MEDITATION: THE FIRE OF TIME

(approx. 10–15 minutes)

This is a meditation that requires you to imagine that you have already died and the body is being burned by the fire of time.[7] It is natural that this idea may cause discomfort. It is helpful to practice this after you have some spent some time exploring the previous two meditations in this chapter. When you are ready, lead yourself through the following steps.

Lie down in a comfortable resting shape. Allow your body to receive and release breath as the navel rises and falls. Hear or mentally repeat the mantra SO HAM (pronounced HUM)—*I am that*—SO as you inhale, HAM as you exhale. Continuing to repeat SO HAM, begin to shape the breath in a 1:2 ratio—for example, inhale four and exhale eight. (10 breaths)

Continue to repeat the mantra SO HAM until the meditation is complete.

Visualize your body as a corpse lying on a wooden platform, surrounded by wood and kindling. Your body is adorned with flowers and dressed in white. Notice the posture of the body and details of the flowers. You may notice family and friends who have gathered. They place flowers on your body. The funeral procession begins and the platform is carried to the water's edge. A fire is lit near the right toe. The fire begins to rise through the body as the funeral pyre is pushed into the water. The fire consumes the entire body and platform. Everything is turned to ash. The winds and waters disperse the ash. The mantra continues to reverberate, as the true Self is not burned but carried by the sound of the mantra, SO HAM.

INTENTIONAL PAUSE

Devote a few minutes to freewriting about your experience of the death meditation and reflecting on the questions below.

- What emotions, sensations or observations did you experience during the meditation?
- What is your essential takeaway from this experience?

COMMUNITY PRACTICE

Cultivate equanimity as you observe the transitions that are happening in your community. Share the tools you have to help with transitions, which might include the death of a community member, the loss of a community space, or change in leadership. Ask yourself, *How can I best be of service to the expansion and nurturing of my community?* Observe resistance to change. Reflect on how this plays out in your life and what lessons you have learned from resisting change. How can you share these lessons in a compassionate way? Questions to ask yourself:

- What is needed at this time? What can I provide?
- Does my Do Word offer any inspiration for how I can be of service to my community in difficult times of change?
- How can I compassionately hold space for whatever is falling away and highlight the need for the collective vision of future possibilities?
- How are happenings in my community circles reflected in the culture at large?

| 9 |

THE ANCESTORS HAVE
YOUR BACK

By venerating the dead we can experience the fullness
of our own souls. Losing touch with these ancestors, we
lose touch with the soul, both theirs and ours.
—*Roshi Joan Halifax*[1]

ONE MORNING I WAS HAVING breakfast with my twelve-year-old
nephew Drew. He looked at me and paused. I knew something interesting
was coming. In a soft voice, he asked, "What was my grandfather, your dad,
like?" I could tell he was relieved when I smiled widely. He seemed to know
this question might cause pain, and I admired his courage in asking. As I was
speaking and sharing a few family memories, I noticed him nodding at certain points as if to say, "That makes sense." I realized he was trying to better
understand *his* dad by asking about his grandfather, who had passed away
when he was three years old.

I was grateful for him asking this question at his age. And as much as I
tried to describe my father, I knew that words could never convey who I saw

and felt him to be the day after he left his body. He was the most brilliant star, floating in the universe, filled with infinite love. As I write this, tears are welling up, and I can feel the pull of *my* personality, the part of me that misses his physical presence and is sad that his life was cut short by Parkinson's and Lewy body dementia. There is still much to heal on the level of the mind. But when I feel with my whole heart and remember the light in his eyes, I feel expansiveness and love. I know that he is still around us, guiding and protecting, just like he did when he was alive. In the twilight of the morning after he transitioned, I was given the gift of knowing that my father's presence in my life is not limited by his physical body.

> Weapons cannot cleave this *atma* (Self), nor fire burn it. Water cannot wet it, nor wind dry it: it is indivisible. It cannot be burnt, not made wet or dry. It is everlasting, all pervading, unchanging stable and eternal.
> —*Bhagavad Gita 2.23–24*[2]

My maternal Nana was a powerful preacher born on a reservation in North Carolina in 1914. She was the leader of her church and a beloved member of her community until her death in 1990. I began to feel her guiding and protective presence when I began teaching yoga in 2001. As my connection to her become more tangible, I became more curious about my other ancestors, especially those who I had never met. At the time, my paternal Bermudian grandmother was still alive, and our family homestead was still intact in Bermuda. But there was scant information about my paternal grandfather, who died three years before I was born. I had only ever seen one picture of him, but I did have one of his possessions—a gold and sapphire signet ring. I created an ancestor altar as a way to remember and honor my lineage, and I placed the ring on the altar. I offered prayers to my ancestors, including the desire for ancestral healing. Once I created a daily ritual of remembering the ancestors, what happened next was magical. I started to receive all kinds of information in the form of long-lost pictures, relatives I didn't know I had emailing me "out of the blue," and new stories from elders that helped to weave a richer picture of my lineage.

INTENTIONAL PAUSE: SELF-INQUIRY

Take a moment to consider the following questions:

- Have you ever felt the "presence" of a loved one (this includes pets) who has passed away, or other energy that you felt was loving, guiding, or protective?
- How did you experience this—sounds, vision, feeling?

WHO ARE THE ANCESTORS?

Once you become curious about ancestors, you have opened the portal to being in relationships with them. Some of us have neglected our ancestors because we have not been taught about their importance. There is power, wisdom, healing, and true wealth in remembering who we are by connecting to the generations that came before us. It is no mistake that when lands were colonized and stolen and people enslaved or persecuted, those people were systematically cut off from their religions, traditions, and family members. When we do not know where and whom we come from, a part of us feels lost and untethered from the greatness of family, culture, and history itself.

We are connected to our ancestors in many ways. Ancestors can be more than just our blood relatives. It was after my Nana transitioned that I learned a family secret. Well, it wasn't so much a family secret but a forgetting. You know the kind—when someone in the family says, "Oh, I can't believe I never told you about that!" I learned that my Nana never had any biological children of her own. She was the second wife of my great-grandfather and had taken my mother and uncle into her home to raise them when their biological mother expressed no desire to do so. So my Nana, who has been guiding me for years, wasn't a blood relative. Is she an ancestor?

Our ancestry moves beyond genealogy, the line of descent traced continuously from one ancestor to the next. When we speak about ancestors in the spiritual sense, our connection to ancestors travels beyond our DNA. Research in the science of epigenetics, which means "above the genes," supports the idea that our environment affects us and that those effects can be passed on to future generations.[3] We have an environmental and blood inheritance from our ancestors. The microbes of an environment should also be considered—the foods our ancestors ate, the places they lived, and the conditions they lived in all make us who we are. And yet we have more than just our family of origin. If we are adopted, our adopted family is also part of our lineage. My Nana was part of my mother's adopted family. Her church, her cooking, her sermons, and even the details she never spoke about, such as growing up on a reservation, are all part of me; she is a powerful ancestor in my lineage.

Our ancestors can include members of our biological family, chosen family, cultural family, and spiritual lineage. The earth itself is our oldest ancestor with whom we have a continuous living relationship. One can only imagine the types of animals and plants our ancestors encountered that are extinct today; they are also ancestors. Acknowledging the ancestors of the land we live on helps us to create a deeper connection with our surrounding as well as honoring the lives and practices of those who came before us.[4] There is no part of the universe to which we are not connected. The earth, the sun, moon, and stars all hold the stories of our ancestors. Ancestral healing and wisdom is a vast tradition beyond the scope of this book; you will find additional resources in the back of the book.[5] Devote a few minutes to answering the following contemplations.

INTENTIONAL PAUSE:
ANCESTOR CONTEMPLATION

- Take a moment to list as many ancestors as possible, including those from any adopted family, chosen family, or spiritual lineages. (For this contemplation, choose those whom you remember fondly and with love.)

- Do you feel connection to any of these ancestors? Have you sensed their presence? If so, how?
- Are there any specific foods or places that connect you with your ancestors? How can you weave these places into your daily life?

HONORING THE GRIEF

Many of our traditional grief rituals are lost to us, which creates a challenge in knowing how to honor ourselves and give ourselves the space needed to heal and grieve those who have passed. There is the pull in Western culture to "get back to normal" and just "get over it." The time of grief holds tremendous power. It is nonlinear and not on the dominant cultural timeline for "moving on." As the pain of loss tenderizes our hearts, it is also our portal for connection. We may pause to remember not only the recently departed but all of those who passed before them. Many prayers and petitions may be offered at this time, and they are heard.

The COVID-19 pandemic brought forward just how unprepared we are as a culture to deal with grief and loss. But it also seemed to propel us into a time when many desired to cultivate a relationship with ancestors and that exploration is becoming more accepted. In times of uncertainty, we intuitively know that a place to turn is the wisdom of our ancestors. As my father was transitioning, I called upon his mother to help greet and guide him on his next journey; this was an instinctual and instant *knowing* of what to do. I believe that download of information came from the ancestral realm, as it wasn't part of my plan for his final day of life. As I landed at the airport after flying overnight, I was told he would be taken to the hospice soon. As we were driving there, I heard a fierce inner voice say, "Do not delay. Go directly to his hospital room. There is very little time." I do not know where that voice came from, but I listened. And those last minutes I spent with him were an initiation into a new way of being present to the continuum of our life force and the power of the true Self.

INTENTIONAL PAUSE: SELF-INQUIRY

Have you ever called upon a deceased relative or friend for guidance or assistance? Describe the circumstances.

REMEMBERING THE ANCESTORS

The urge to move on with life after the loss of a loved one should not be in trying to get back to normal. What we once knew as "normal" is in the past. But moving on can mean exploring a deepening in life that includes a relationship with ancestors. Indigenous traditions speak of the ills that can befall us when we forget to honor our ancestors. The Pueblo people of the Southwest believe that when we forget to honor our ancestors, the rains will cease to fall.[6] To the Dagara people in West Africa, "veneration of the ancestors is so ingrained in daily life that forgetting them is either an act of carelessness or willful disengagement."[7] Even if we have never been taught to honor our ancestors, there is part of us that knows and remembers. To some of us in the West, having a relationship with our ancestors feels scary and uncomfortable. We've been peppered with images and movies of the paranormal, ghosts, and the "dangerous" voodoo witch doctor who primes us to fear our inheritance. And then there is the reality that not all of our ancestors were good people.

Yoli Maya Yeh is an educator in comparative religions and global studies who works at the intersection of indigenous preservation, healing arts, and social justice. Raised in her family's Native American spiritual teachings, Yoli had a vision decades ago that led her to lead work on ancestral remembrance. "It would seem that our forgetting of honoring the ancestors as a cultural practice was greatly accelerated by industrialization," she says. "We know these systems are designed to separate us from nature and to make us think we are individual, disembodied, and alone."[8]

Taking small steps to honor and remember the ancestors is a practice that we can weave into daily life, or practice on special occasions. Daily rituals can also support practices that you may already have as a part of your ancestral remembrance, like lighting yahrzeit candles or celebrating Día de los Muertos.

PRACTICES TO CONNECT WITH THE ANCESTORS

The following are simple practices you can do to honor your ancestors. Devote time after each ritual or practice to answer the self-inquiry questions and to journal or freewrite. You will also find other resources to explore on page 184.

ANCESTOR ALTAR

Create a small altar to honor your ancestors.

The altar can be as simple or extravagant as you wish.

If you have any images of the ancestors you would like to honor, place them on the altar. Just make sure you are not in the pictures.

You can also add personal items such as jewelry, glasses, car keys, or handwritten notes.

If you know your ancestors' favorite foods, you can leave these offerings on special occasions, such as birthdays and anniversaries.

If you do not have personal items or pictures or know who your ancestors were, find out what kind of crops were grown in the region of the world where your ancestors are from and place those seeds on the altar.

Place a small vessel of water on the space that you choose for the ancestor altar. The element of water is important for the ancestors in many traditions as this is how the ancestors travel to the ancestor realm. Water is sacred for prayers and purification and represents the divinity of life. Add a stick of incense or sacred smoke from the indigenous land of your ancestors

Take a moment each day to light a candle or incense and remember those who came before you. Keep the altar clean, and refresh it often with fresh water. Offer prayers for the healing of your ancestors.

ANCESTOR NEW MOON PRACTICE[9]

Each new moon, take a few minutes to sit in front of the ancestor altar and meditate. Be open.

This is a time to remember and name your ancestors. The new moon represents a time of new beginnings, transition, liminal space, and the ancestral world.

Begin with your maternal lineage, naming all of those whose names you know in order of most recent to oldest. (Remember that ancestors include blood lineage, chosen family, and spiritual family.) Move on to your paternal line, saying the names out loud in the same way. You may prefer to continue by including your chosen family, spiritual lineage, the ancestors of all of your lifetimes, and especially the countless ancestors whose names we will never know.

If you choose to, this can be a time for you to connect more deeply with your ancestors by asking questions or to receive guidance and inspiration. Once again, be open to messages and how they may appear. Take a few minutes to sit quietly in front of the altar with your awareness drawn inward. Draw a circle of energetic protection around yourself. Around that protective circle of light, feel the presence of your elevated ancestors—those who are well in spirit and have your best interests at heart. Feel them gathering around the circumference of the circle. Their presence cleanses the space outside of the circle, and you sense a force of protection and healing. Whatever questions or guidance you need, ask for it in your own way, with reverence and love. When you feel complete with the meditation, devote several minutes to freewriting, describing your experience with words, images, or whatever helps you to capture the essence of your time in meditation. As the days move on and the moon becomes more illuminated, continue to be aware that guidance can come in many forms. Stay awake to subtle energies, dreams, and synchronicities.

ANCESTOR YOGA NIDRA

(approx. 20–25 minutes)

The practice of yoga nidra is a profoundly restful yet spiritually awakening practice of sustaining consciousness in the liminal space between sleeping and waking.

Begin by bringing awareness to your heart center, deep behind your sternum in the center of your chest. Bring your attention to your heart with a deep, deep, deep breath in; and with the exhale, release an audible sweet sigh out. (9 times total)

Inhale at your heart center; exhale.

Each time you exhale, feel as though you are releasing anything weighing heavy on your heart. Feel it releasing through the back of your heart space. Feel it releasing and being received by the earth. (9 times)

Bring your awareness to your navel and notice that your body is breathing. As you notice that your body is receiving an inhale, just feel your navel rising. Notice that your body is releasing an exhale, and feel your navel fall. Feel as though all your breath is moving in your belly. As you inhale, your navel expands. Exhale, your navel contracts.

Notice that with each breath your chest becomes more and more still. For the next nine breaths, feel your breath moving in your belly. You don't need to make anything happen; just notice the movement of your belly.

Feel the earth beneath your body, or whatever it is that you are lying on, and as your body receives an inhale, sense the earth as it rises up to hold and cradle your body. As you exhale, you release and let go into that hold. As your body receives an inhale, the earth rises up to hold and cradle your body. As you exhale, your body releases. Observe the earth rising up, and feel yourself softening into the earth as your body exhales. (9 breaths)

Feel yourself dropping deeper and deeper into the hold of the earth. As you continue to drop deeper with every exhale, draw a circle of protective light around your body. Trust the presence of this protective light, and draw another circle of light around that circle—a circle of healing. Continue to allow your body to drop in deeper, and draw one more circle of light around the circle of healing—a circle of wisdom. Feel all the protective forces of your guides, elevated ancestors, and benevolent beings around the circle. Feel the presence of divine wisdom, protection, and healing.

With each breath, you receive support rising up from the earth beneath you, but you feel and sense the support drawing in from the sides, from above you, from below you. The space around your body is completely supported and protected. You are in the center of the circles. All sounds, thoughts, and concerns are on the outside of the circles.

Count your breaths backward from 27. Silently repeat to yourself, inhaling 27, exhaling 27, inhaling 26, and exhaling 26. Keep going on your own until you reach zero. Each breath allows you to release a layer of constriction and a layer of thought. When you arrive at zero, the body and mind feel free. If you lose your place in counting down, start back at 27 again. (1 minute)

When you arrive at zero, let go of the counting. Become aware that there is a force outside of you that is compelling you to breathe. The prayers and wisdom of your ancestors ride on every breath. Let your awareness rest on that stream of unending wisdom and love that is compelling you to breathe. Feel the breath being received from infinity and returning to infinity. (1 minute)

The space above is holding you. The earth below is holding you. The ancestors are protecting you. Every breath offers an opportunity for remembrance to unfold. Feel and sense the inner space of your body as a dark night's sky. The space inside your body is a dark night's sky. The space outside of your body is a dark night's sky, only separated by your skin. Let awareness rest in the dark night sky inside of the body.

Rest attention at your third-eye point. At your third-eye point, see a tiny point of blue starlight twinkling. At your throat center, see a tiny blue starlike point of light twinkling. At every place that I mention in your body, you'll see this tiny blue starlike point of light twinkling in the dark night sky of your body. Right shoulder joint—tiny blue starlike point of light. Right elbow joint. Right wrist joint. Tip of your right thumb. Tip of your second finger. Tip of your third finger. Tip of your fourth finger. Tip of your pinkie finger. Right wrist joint. Right elbow joint. Right shoulder joint. Pit of your throat—tiny blue starlike point of light. Left shoulder joint. Left elbow joint. Left wrist joint. Tip of youre left thumb. Tip of your second finger. Tip of your third finger. Tip of your fourth finger. Tip of your pinkie finger. Left wrist joint. Left elbow joint. Left shoulder joint. Pit of your throat. Center of your chest. Right side of your chest. Left side of your chest. Center of your chest. Navel center. Pelvic center. Right hip joint. Right knee joint—tiny blue starlike point of light. Right ankle joint. Tip of your right big toe. Tip of your second toe. Tip of your third toe. Tip of your fourth toe. Tip of your pinkie toe. Right ankle joint. Right knee joint. Right hip joint. Pelvic center. Left hip joint. Left knee joint. Left ankle joint. Tip of your left big toe. Tip of your second toe. Tip of your third toe. Tip of your fourth toe. Tip of your pinkie toe. Left ankle joint. Left knee joint. Left hip joint. Pelvic center. Navel center. Center of your chest, deep behind your sternum. Throat center. Third-eye point. See all of these tiny blue starlike points of light, twinkling inside your body like a constellation of stars.

Now, as if those stars were reflecting light into a night sky above your body, see the constellation of stars directly above your body, to the right of your body, to the left of your body, above and below. Remember the stars twinkling inside of your body.

Feel as though you are floating in a sea of starlight. Feel all of the starlight from both inside and outside of your body descend into your spiritual heart center. Your entire heart space is filled with radiant light, like a sea of liquid diamonds.

Let your body soften in the presence of this light, the light of the ancestors. Feel as though the light and wisdom of your ancestors and guides are guiding you deeper and deeper into the space of your heart, to a space where you will find a cave.

Let wisdom and intuition guide you to the door of this cave.

When you reach the door of this cave, push the door open, and there you will see a central fire, a central flame. It is that eternal flame that is that place within you that knows both the cause and the cure. This flame is the hearth of both your lineage and your power.

You see a figure sitting in a cross-legged position in front of that fire. As you walk closer, you take your seat in front of that fire and sit in front of that being. As you sit in front of this being, you sense that this being is the future ancestor that lives within you.

Gaze into the eyes of yourself as the future ancestor. Do not look away from their gaze.

Continue to look into their eyes and notice what you feel, sense, or see.

Begin to sense the rhythm of their breath.

As they exhale, you sense, see, or feel a stream of rose-colored light releasing from their nostrils.

Your breaths begin to synchronize. As they breathe out this rose-colored light, you breathe that light in; and as you exhale rose-colored light, they breathe that light in.

You are sharing breath with them as you gaze into their eyes. For the next two minutes, share this breath of rose-colored light with yourself as a future ancestor.

As you continue to share this breath, in the form of a petition or a prayer or a request, ask for anything that you need in your life right now. (1 minute)

The future ancestor has a gift for you, but first they would like you to place anything in the fire that no longer serves you—anything that is holding you back, any ways of being, any beliefs, any old baggage. They ask you now to offer this into the fire as a way to empower your strength and your wisdom.

Take the next few minutes to make that offering into the fire. Anything that no longer serves you, make an offering to your own power, to your own future.

They want you to know that you can always come back to this hearth, back to this fire, to make an offering, to receive any wisdom.

Feel them coming close; listen closely as they lean into your right ear and whisper a message.

Once you have received the message, they will present you with a gift.

Receive their gift.

Now together, you both lie on the cave floor and rest, let go of all doing. (3 minutes)

As the practice comes to a close, allow your body to be as still as possible and feel yourself in the space in between, the liminal. Remember the message and the gift. Hold them close as you begin to feel the light outside the cave door becoming brighter. As you deepen your breath, you resurface to the waking state. Begin to move your body gently, and in your own way come back to being seated. Dedicate some time to freewriting and answering the following self-inquiry questions once you feel grounded.

SELF-INQUIRY

- What gift or message did you receive? What significance do they hold for you?
- How can you live into being a good future ancestor? What karmic patterns have been handed down through your lineage (blood or adopted) that you would like to release?
- What generational wealth in the form of stories, rituals, recipes, relationships with elders, or tending to land and home are you ready to reclaim?

Write, draw, or make notes about anything else that feels meaningful.

When you honor the ancestor field you honor yourself. When you honor yourself you honor the ancestor field. You are so very special as you are the living ancestor.

—*Yoli Maya Yeh*

COMMUNITY PRACTICE

Consider how you can practice ancestral remembrance within your community.

- Offer to hold space for friends and community when someone dear passes on. Be ready to show up with presence in a way you may never have before.
- Make an offering in your own way in honor of someone in the community who has passed on. Make it meaningful, going to a special place you know they loved and leaving a flower mandala, pouring libations, dancing to their favorite song, or offering flowers to a body of water. Rituals of honoring can be done in a communal gathering or on your own.
- Remember birthdays and anniversaries. Share stories.

| 10 |

DREAM WISDOM

As you work with your dreams, you will become aware of
your own "soul" or "Higher Self" or "inner Light."
—*Swami Sivananda Radha*[1]

INDIGENOUS CULTURES, ARTISTS, and inventors have long known
and revered the power of the dream. Dreams are the messengers of spiritual
insights, prophecies, and creative inspiration—a doorway to discovering
more about what lies in the depths of our being.[2] Some cultures and traditions believe that dreams are portals to other realms of existence, dimensions,
or worlds. Paying attention to our dreaming life is a way of weaving practice
into the full cycle of a day and honoring the states consciousness that we
usually dismiss as "not real" or unimportant. *Svapna* (dream state)[3] is one
of the four states of consciousness, and dreaming is what those in the know
refer to as "night school." The great Indian philosopher, teacher, and poet Sri
Aurobindo said that "sadhana can go on in the dream or sleep state as well as
in the waking" and that dreams can "convey great truths that are not so easy
to get in the waking state."[4]

When we are ready to explore dreams as a valid source of knowledge, we should ask ourselves a few questions: *Who is the one that is dreaming? Where do I go when I dream? Is the dream a real place?* I am not sure that we will ever scientifically know the answers, and maybe they are not meant to be known. But if we can learn to embrace our dreams as a significant part of our lives and not something to ignore, a window to something magical opens. We initiate a relationship with an unknown and mystical part of ourselves—the dreaming self.

PANDEMIC DREAMS

During the pandemic I noticed that my dreams became more vivid and seemed to be filled with more messages, symbols, and what I interpreted as sacred instructions. I began to craft my online offerings in alignment with some of the messages that I was receiving from the dream world, which mostly had to do with the importance of community, ancestors, and the kind of practices that would be helpful in the time of uncertainty. As I began to share my dreams with some of my peers, we noticed similarities in our dreaming content. It seemed that we were often swirling in a collective dream. The message was clear: don't fall asleep to the world, stay awake in the states of consciousness, and remember the wisdom of the dreams.

The pandemic affected dreams for many of us. Scientists found that the closer people were to the epicenter of the pandemic—health-care workers, for example—the more their dreams had to do with the virus itself.[6] What we chose to do with our time in isolation may also have affected our dream world. Were we practicing more meditation and yoga? Were we resting and spending time in nature? Were we binging on streaming services, social media, and the news? People recognized that their dreams were becoming so bizarre that the hashtag #coronadreams began to trend on Twitter. It may have been the first time in history that we collectively started to pay attention to our dreams and then publicly share them. The first important point of entry to dreamwork is making a commitment to cultivate a relationship with your dreams. Be intentional and imagine dreamwork to be like a courtship with a mysterious aspect of yourself that is illusive yet powerful and revealing. If you are someone who often has nightmares, set a clear intention to focus on something positive and loving before going to sleep. The more we create intentions to remember our dreams and to record what we remember, the more our dreams may reveal themselves to us. It is a wonderful practice to enter this journey toward dream wisdom with a sense of curiosity and devotion inspired by bhakti yoga. Bhakti is the yoga of devotion; it is the practice of seeing the Divine in everything. All too often we are tempted to use our practices to extract, manifest, and become more powerful in a hierarchal way. Remember that attachment to *siddhis*, or "special powers," is an obstacle to liberation.[7] Instead, as you cultivate this relationship with your dreaming self and begin to explore the Divine within you through the world of dreams, be open and let go of the need to figure things out from the level of the mind.

SELF-INQUIRY

Consider the following questions:

- How would you describe your relationships with dreams?
- Has there been any point in your life where there was a drastic change in how you dreamed or your ability to remember your dreams? If so, was there any transition in your life that correlates to this time?
- As you recall your history of dreaming life, what dream stands out as being the most profound? Describe the dream in detail, including when it occurred and why it was so important.
- What were your dreams like during the early stages of the COVID-19 pandemic? How did they transform and shift over time?

NINE-DAY DREAM SADHANA

Exploring a dream practice consistently for nine consecutive nights might be helpful. To begin, you will need a dream journal—a simple journal kept by your bedside dedicated to transcribing your dreams. Each night you will do the following:

- Name your truest desire for wanting to connect with the realm of dreams. Examples might be "to know my true Self" or "to explore other realms." As you enter the practice, soften trying to make anything happen and be open to the magic of exploring your dreams.
- When you are ready to go to sleep, let your attention rest in your throat center. As you rest attention at your throat, feel, sense, or imagine a full bright moon resting at your throat center. (3 breaths) Sense that breath is moving in and out of your throat center. Silently repeat to yourself, *Tonight I will remember my dreams* while keeping awareness at your throat center, imagining the full, bright moon. (3 breaths)
- Allow yourself to fall asleep. It is very rare that we remember dreams from the first part of the night when we are in non-REM sleep. The second part of the night and hour or so before waking is mostly REM sleep. The dream yoga teacher Andrew Holecek calls the forty-five minutes to an hour before waking "prime-time dreamtime."[8]
- Wake up without an alarm clock. Either rise naturally with the sun or use the Mental Alarm Clock Practice (see page 163) to awaken in the morning.
- As soon as you feel yourself in the space between sleeping and waking,[9] allow yourself to be perfectly still for a time, especially your head. Try to recall the dreams from the night before. You just need one thread of the dream to begin.
- When you are ready to move and have a thread of the dream to pull forward, begin to transcribe it in your dream journal. It doesn't have to be a long paragraph—perhaps just a word, color, feeling, or image from the

dream; add as many details as you have. If you do not have any memory of the dream, note that as well. Make a note of the quality of your mind, mood, emotions, or thoughts upon waking as well.

- Begin to categorize your dreams. In this stage, you want to divest from looking for information from others. Plenty of books offer meanings of dream symbols and the categories of dreams, but this is where you want to connect with your own inner wisdom. Create your own descriptions for types of dreams. Examples might be "spiritual," "prophetic," "scary," "recurring," "healing," or "magical." Each morning, note the type of dream. If you start looking for symbols in a book, you will likely find more than one meaning depending on the source. Each culture has a different relationship with a symbol or image. For instance, a Pentecostal preacher may have a different reaction to a snake appearing in a dream than someone from a Hindu background. Let the meaning unfold within you over the nine days.
- Once you have completed the nine-day practice, review your dream journal and notice any themes. Notice if you intuit any meaning coming forth. Are these dreams just the mind processing information of the day? Did you receive a message or creative inspiration or enter another realm?

DREAMING TEMPLE RITUAL

Prepare yourself for bed and find your comfortable resting shape. Have a journal by your bedside.

Bring awareness to the center of your forehead and feel that space softening. Each exhale allows the space at the center of your forehead to soften. (1 minute)

Begin to notice your navel rising on the inhale and falling on the exhale. Let go of trying to shape or control your breath in any way and just notice your navel rising and falling. (5 breaths)

Now bring awareness to the top of your head. Feel as though your breath is moving in through the top of your head as your body inhales and exhales through your pelvic center or womb space. (3 times)

Inhale through the top of your head, and exhale through your navel. (3 times)

Inhale through the top of your head, and exhale through your heart center. (3 times)

Inhale through the top of your head, and exhale through your throat center. (3 times)

Inhale through the top of your head, and exhale through the third-eye point. (3 times)

Now begin to descend awareness through the centers again, this time with one breath each.

Inhale through the top of your head. Exhale through your throat center, seeing a full bright moon in your throat center. (1 breath)

Inhale through the top of your head. Exhale through your heart center. (1 breath)

Let your awareness rest at your heart center. Remember the full moon resting at your throat, and feel the rays of moonlight illuminating your heart center. This illumination guides a way to a path that leads to a doorway. Follow the path and pause at the doorway.

As you push that door open, it reveals a beautiful lake. You remember that you are in a sacred place.

You take a sip from this pristine, cold mountain lake and anoint your body with this water. As you anoint your body, you begin to hear the sound of OM chanted in the distance.

You hear temple bells ringing. Begin to walk on the path that leads to this temple.

As you walk along this path, you notice that there are wildflowers growing and all manner of creatures wandering the land.

Eventually you arrive at the temple steps. Now notice the steps to the temple. The steps are fairly steep. You slowly make your way up these steps. One by one. There are 54 steps. And as you enter the temple doors, you start to notice that the sound of AUM becomes louder. You feel the vibration in all of the sacred centers of your body

You open the door to the temple, and in the temple you see that there is an altar space. At the altar space, you notice that there is a single flame on the altar. But the altar needs to be cleaned. Begin to clear and clean the altar. Light a stick of incense or sacred smoke.

Take your comfortable seat in front of the altar, offer any prayers, and make any requests to the sacred fire. Begin to feel your body becoming very heavy. You are ready to take sacred rest. Notice a small, simple resting nest near the altar and take rest there. Allow yourself to now fall asleep and enter the dream space. When the time comes for you to awaken, be as still as possible. You will hear the sound of AUM. Remembering that you are in the temple. You will follow the path back to the lake and then to the door of your heart. Hover in this in-between space as long as possible. Transcribe your memory of the dream fragments in your journal.

SELF-INQUIRY

Devote several minutes to remembering your experience with the practice.

- What did you see, feel, or sense during your experience?
- What happened when you came back to the waking state?
- As you left the temple, did you remember the way back to the lake and doorway?

HERBS TO SUPPORT DREAMING

Different herbs can assist in the potency of dreaming and dreaming recall. Before introducing any new herbs, please consult a doctor about potential allergies, other contraindications, or interactions with medications or supplements you should avoid. Try to access these herbs from a fresh and trusted source, such as a local herbalist or apothecary.

- Mugwort—dried, can be placed in a sachet under your pillow; as an oil, rubbed on your temples and the back of your neck; as a sacred incense, can be burned before sleeping
- African dream root (*Silene undulata*)—usually made as tincture
- Blue lotus tea (*Nelumbo nucifera*)—relaxing; produces vivid dreams
- Passionflower tea—relaxing; produces vivid dreams
- Chaparral tincture—said to have the effect of cleansing things buried in the psyche

PRACTICES TO SUPPORT DREAMING

- Meditations focusing on the third-eye center
- Yoga nidra practices with focus on a full moon at your throat center (the center of dreaming)
- Dream journaling—the practice of translating anything you can remember from your dreams (e.g., a color, image, sound, person, feeling, or fragrance)
- Daydreaming—allowing yourself to have spaciousness of time, thought, imagination without a specific goal; just letting the mind wander to be free and creative, and allowing any narratives or images to unfurl naturally and without judgment
- Creative practices—undertaking a new creative practice such as painting, poetry, singing, or playing an instrument which wakes up new neural pathways in the brain
- Silence—devoting thirty minutes to be in silence before bed; no phones, books, or writing, just sitting in silence
- Learning about the crone goddess Dhumavati, who represents the void state of meditation, and Swapneshwari, the goddess of dreams

COMMUNITY CARE

Share your dreams with those who you share a home with or in community. Join a dream circle. You may be surprised at synchronicities and how messages and information from your dreams support and inform each other. If you have a dream that seems important about a member of your community or family, share it with them. The dream may not seem to be of significance to you, but it may hold special meaning and wisdom for someone else. We never know when we have been chosen to carry a message from the dream realm.

The dream expert Chanti Tacoronte-Perez shares dream rituals in community. "Sharing dreams is ancient medicine," she says. "Community dreaming allows one to acknowledge pain, discomfort, fear, emotions, and images that may be difficult to talk about in waking reality. Draped by the dream state, challenging, provocative, nightmare-like experiences find their voice and are allies in witnessing and processing grief and acknowledging joy. . . . Sharing your dreams is also a powerful act of self-expression which pushes against hierarchal-colonial systems that attempt to diminish one's connection to intuition, imagination, creativity, and critical thinking. In other words, community dreaming, which tends to the collective dream, can rebalance circular wisdom while living in a linear world."[10]

| 11 |

YOU ARE LUMINOUS,
WE ARE LUMINOUS

IN THE WINTER OF 2007, I was preparing to leave the small Northern California town I had been calling home. Five years earlier, I had convinced my company to let me work remotely part-time. It was a way to transition from the toxic environment of Hollywood film production to a life I dreamed of living deep in nature, sharing yoga, and independently producing films only when I was inspired. I thought I had left the grind behind, but everything was about to change. My marriage had fallen apart, though it was never really together in the first place. The economy was in crisis; my donation-run yoga studio was suffering. I couldn't concentrate on the film I had just produced, and I realized life in this small town would not be sustainable. I was at the most significant crossroads of my life.

My yoga practice and nature were the only things holding me together. I decided to go to a small ashram in Grass Valley, about a three-hour drive from my home. Aside from the small nine-person volunteer staff, I was the only guest on the eighty-acre campus. One of the staff asked me what I would like to choose for my daily *seva*. *Seva* means "thread" or "selfless service"—the spiritual practice of doing acts of love and kindness without the agenda of personal gain. Seva is an act born of divine love and is part of the paths of karma (action) and bhakti (devotion). I chose kitchen duty, my *least* favorite activity in the world, hoping it would create some kind of *tapas* (inner heat) and move me out of feeling stuck.

My stay at the ashram was a healing balm. I spent much of my time in silence, walking in nature and meditating. I joined the staff for meals and morning kirtan, journaled, and practiced gentle yoga asana twice daily. As the days went by, I noticed I was beginning to look forward to kitchen duty. I saw how much joy and pride the people cooking the food exuded. They watched everyone taking their first bites of the meal with huge smiles. You could feel the love they had for being of service. I was a part of a community, doing my part to support the whole. It was the remembrance that I needed to begin my healing journey; it wasn't about what I was doing, but *how* I was doing it. When I had two days left in my stay, one of the staff told me, "Two more people are coming. You won't be alone anymore!" Later in the day, I saw a van pull up with two bearded men in their early twenties; we waved from afar, quickly introduced ourselves, and then went about our day.

It had been my practice for years (and still is) to rise before the sun to meditate and chant the Surya Gayatri mantra as the sun rises. The Surya Gayatri is a mantra I have chanted thousands of times. Vamadeva David Frawley describes it as representing the "transformational power inherent in the sun, not only to change night into day but also to take us beyond the darkness of the ego into the infinite light of the higher Self."[1]

That morning after finishing my chanting, I walked in silence toward the kitchen and opened the door. Brilliant sunlight was flooding through the window. Just at that moment, I experienced a flood of light emanating from my heart center back to the streaming sunlight, an endless wave of golden light. I was watching everything unfold as if I was outside of my body, a passive observer. Then I noticed one of the bearded men standing at the sink. In silence, the man turned toward me and smiled; the light enveloped us both with this blissful feeling of love, joy, and oneness. Our hearts connected, no separation between us. A sense of deep recognition came over me. I *knew* this soul of pure love, light, and joy. We shared the same essence of light within us. We never exchanged a single word. What seemed like time standing still was only a minute or so. I had tasted and seen something true inside of me. Was it because of my practice? Was it because of the bearded man, the sunlight, nature, silence? I will never know. I only saw him once more before I left. I decided not to say a word; we just gave each other a knowing nod. Not everything sacred needs to be talked about right away. It takes time to process and integrate. I realized that my small self, having that experience, may have said, *It's love at first sight. You need to do something; this is the answer to healing your heartbreak!* But no, another part of me was awake to this experience; it had higher intelligence and discernment than my thinking mind. For whatever reason, at that moment my ego was sleeping, and I was awake to something real.

The experience reminded me of that moment of presence that I experienced thirteen years before on my balcony in South Africa. That moment led me to yoga, and the moment I just described has fueled my continuous practice and sharing of yoga. When I returned home, my ex was there clearing out his things and getting ready to move in with his new girlfriend. I still carried the experience in my cells as I walked through the door. He looked at me puzzled and said, "What do you have to be so happy about?" Without thinking, the answer came out of my mouth: "My joy is not dependent on you or any outside circumstances." I surprised myself with this knowing. I did not even feel like I was the one speaking the words. I had a new understanding of what it meant to be me, beyond my personality. There really was a place within me that was beyond all sorrow.[2]

In my life since then, I try to remember this, and there have been many times when I have forgotten. I often come back to practices to help me remember what my soul already knows. Healing is full of ebbs and flows between remembering and forgetting, releasing and gripping, doubting and knowing. It has been my experience that when I sustain a thread of practice through the days, life is filled with more Self-remembrance, love, and joy.

Feelings of despair, powerlessness, and instability can arise when we forget that pure light, love, and joy is our birthright. Learning to rest in our joy is counterculture. It's time we remember joy as part of our innate essence and incorporate the things that bring us joy into our daily life. The following practice is a way to anchor yourself in joy. Find a quiet and comfortable place to practice and have your journal with you.

RECLAIMING JOY PRACTICE

(approx. 10–15 minutes)

You can find audio of this practice at www.shambhala.com/TheLuminousSelf Practices.

Find a comfortable meditation shape.

Close your eyes or soften your gaze.

Scan your body, noticing any tension you may be holding.

Notice where you can soften tension in your body. Feel the center of your forehead soften, your eyes and eyebrows soften, and your jaw, throat, shoulders, and hips. Notice any other parts of your body that would like to soften. (2 minutes)

Begin to feel your spine as the central axis of your body. Notice the space to the left of your spine, to the right of your spine, above your spine, and below your spine. Sense all of the space that your body occupies. (1 minute)

Become aware that your body is breathing. Feel the flow of your breath as it moves in through your nostrils. Feel the moment your breath touches your nostrils; follow its path as it moves in through your nostrils, riding up the roof of your nose toward your third-eye center. Your breath moves from your third-eye center back out through your nostrils. (1 minute)

Continue to notice and sense this breath moving in this way. Feel your breath moving in through your nostrils toward the third-eye center, the midway point between your eyebrows. Breath moves back out through your nostrils. (1 minute)

Begin to feel, sense, or trust your breath as two streams of white light. This light moves through both nostrils to your third-eye point, meeting at the third eye and then moving back out as your body exhales from your third-eye point. Notice these two streams of breath like an inverted V of light. Sense, feel, or trust that prana, the vital life force, is riding on the breath as light. (2 minutes)

Now feel and sense your third-eye point. Feel as though there is light that has been collected there. Notice the vibration of a collected pool of light. (1 minute)

The light begins to move. Guided by divine intelligence, it moves downward toward the center of your chest, deep behind your breastbone. Allow your attention to rest at the center of your chest. (1 minute)

Remember a moment of joy. A moment of pure joy, pure bliss and freedom. Allow yourself to remember moments of joy. Let your mind move from one moment to another. See where you were, what you were doing, feel what it felt like in your body—complete joy and freedom. See, feel, remember these moments of joy. (2 minutes)

Allow yourself to rest in one moment of joy—one moment of joy that feels potent. If you feel as though you can't find a moment of joy or remember a moment of joy, imagine what a moment of joy would feel like. (1 minute)

As you're in this moment of joy, begin to feel it permeate the entire body. Feel it in every cell of your body. As you breathe in, you feel as though you are breathing in this moment of joy, and as you exhale, you breathe out this vibration of joy. Feel as though the pores in your body have opened, and they are receiving the joy as an inhale and releasing the joy as your body exhales. Remember yourself beyond your personality. Remember yourself as joy. (1 minute)

Bring your awareness and all of the energy of joy back to your third-eye point. See a blank movie screen in front of your closed eyes. Project that energy of joy onto the movie screen and see a joyful life projected in front of you. Sense what life will be like if you reclaimed joy. As you close the practice silently say to yourself three times, *I reclaim joy. I am joy. Joy is my true nature.*

Come back slowly.

INTENTIONAL PAUSE

If you saw any image or colors or felt anything about reclaiming joy, devote a few moments to writing in your journal about it.

- What moment of joy did you choose?
- What did you see in this space of your closed eyes, as a projection of what life can be like if you choose to remember and reclaim your joy?

THE LUMINOUS EGG

The cosmic egg is an image that symbolizes creation in many cultures. The egg can represent infinite potential in the form of the unmanifest waiting to come into creation. In yogic teachings, the cosmic egg is known as *hiranyagarbha*, the "golden or universal womb." Hiranyagarbha is said to be the original teacher of yoga.[3] Inside each of us there is said to be a golden place, a seed of light that contains the entire universe.[4] When we realize the true Self, our individual consciousness is joined with the universal consciousness. This is the union referred to in the translation of the word *yoga*—"to yoke." Imagine if everyone in the world who is "doing yoga" could explore a different understanding of the word. What would the world of "wellness" transform into?

LUMINOUS SELF YOGA NIDRA

(approx. 15–20 minutes)

You can find audio of this practice at www.shambhala.com/TheLuminousSelf Practices. This practice is inspired by the teachings of Swami Veda Bharati's three-minute yoga nidra, the Himalayan Tradition practice of Aharana, and personal practices and experiences of the luminous egg..

Begin by practicing tension and relaxation by tensing and releasing your body's muscles. Make fists with your hands; tighten your arm muscles, your legs, your belly, your face, your buttocks, and every muscle in your body. And then release. (3 times)

Let your body release into the support beneath you. Find a comfortable resting position for your body, supported by whatever props you need. Let the shape of your body feel nurtured and supported.

Notice that your body is breathing. Feel your navel moving up and down effortlessly as you receive your breath. Feel the abundance available to you through this effortless breath. (10 breaths)

Continue to feel the support of the earth beneath you. Notice how when your body breathes in, the earth feels as though it is rising up to hold you, offering a healing space for you to rest. As your body exhales, you soften into the kindness and compassion of the earth. Experience unconditional holding, nurturing, and love. Body inhales, the earth rises. Body exhales, soften into the support beneath you.

Welcome the permission to receive all of what the earth has to offer. (10 breaths)

Devote the next three breaths to offering your gratitude back to the earth.

Rest your attention at your forehead. Feel your forehead softening. The center of your forehead is softening. Sense your breath penetrating deeply into that space of your forehead, as though it is smoothing out and softening any wrinkles on the surface of your skin and deeper into your mind. (5 breaths)

Travel through your body and feel one breath at each of the following places. One breath in and out—just natural breath letting go of controlling or forcing.

Feel your breath at your third-eye point. At your eyes and eyebrows. Bridge of your nose. Cheeks and jaw. Throat center. Heart center. Solar plexus. Navel center. Pelvic center. Base of your spine. Hips. Knees. Ankles. Tips of your toes. Sense three breaths moving in and out from the tips of your toes. Soles of your feet. Heels. Ankles. Hips. Base of your spine. Pelvic center. Navel center. Heart center. Throat center. Shoulder joints. Upper arms. Elbows. Wrists. Fingertips. Feel three breaths moving in and out from your fingertips. Elbows. Shoulders. Throat center. Third-eye point. Forehead. For three breaths, move in and out of the forehead.

Feel your body being held by the earth.

For the next minute, just feel your body being fully supported and held by the earth. (1 minute)

Rest attention at your third-eye point. (1 minute)

Rest at your throat center and feel or sense the presence of a full, bright moon. Resting at your throat center. Healing. Moonlight. (2 minutes)

Rest awareness at your heart center. At the center of your heart, sense the presence of a golden flame. Notice this flame in the shape of a golden egg. (1 minute)

Inside of this golden egg is a tiny version of you. Lying down. Resting. You are cocooned in a place of protection. A place where you have permission to experience your true Self. See and feel yourself resting inside of this golden egg. (3 minutes)

Remember yourself inside of this golden egg. Notice as you inhale, this golden egg is becoming larger. With each natural breath, the golden egg becomes larger and larger. Eventually it fully encompasses your physical body. Continue to rest here, your whole physical body now inside of the golden egg. (1 minute)

Continue to feel this golden healing light. Feel and sense that this light frequency is healing and uniquely calibrates itself to you. (3 minutes)

Now for the next three minutes, let go of all doing; just be. (3 minutes)

Slowly begin to awaken from the practice when you are ready, gently moving and deepening the breath. Only when you are ready.

INTENTIONAL PAUSE

Devote five to ten minutes to journal, draw, or freewrite about your experience.

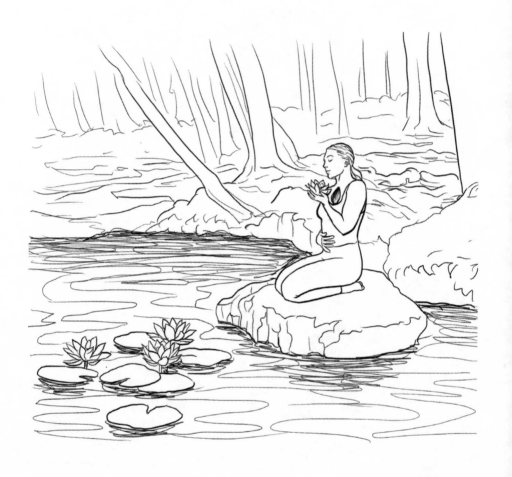

CONCLUSION: INITIATE
YOURSELF—RITUALS OF POWER

WE ARE ALWAYS IN TRANSITION but not often awake to all the liminal space we encounter. *Liminal* refers to being between or at a threshold. When we are at a threshold, we leave one space behind and enter another, allowing us to pause and be present. In that pause we can choose to remember what heals, inspires, and nurtures us and what we want to leave behind. In every transition, we consciously or unconsciously choose what we are bringing forward. We experience transitions in every moment—the space between breaths, sunrise and sunset, the space of falling asleep and waking. You can honor some of these natural transitional spaces of the day by chanting a mantra, lighting incense, sipping tea, journaling, or taking full-moon ritual baths. Maybe you have already created new personal rituals as you have moved through this book and explored the inquiries, practices, and contemplations.

In many cultures, big threshold moments are recognized with rites of passage or initiation ceremonies. Because many of us have lost connection with our ancestral roots, left spiritual lineages because of abuse, or do not have relationships with our elders, we have lost the remembrance of how to honor the power of life's threshold moments. And sometimes *we* need to create the threshold.

A threshold moment for me was when I realized the power that being attacked on the school bus and having eggs cracked over my head held over me decades later. I was afraid of being seen. I was fearful of being successful, and I was scared of being in a community. At one point during a yoga class, I realized that this moment from the past was what caused me to obsessively pull out my hair. I was ready to stop bringing the past forward and was able to stop this harmful behavior by becoming more present. But that wasn't enough. I needed to create a pause—an intentional threshold to healing.

I needed a ritual, an initiation, to mark the moment that I decided to leave the past pain behind and move forward in a way that was informed by the past without being a prisoner to it.

As I considered a ritual for myself, I understood the power was in the egg; the smeared yolk of the egg over my dark skin was a symbol of shame. And I had been carrying it around for long enough. I needed to transform the egg into a symbol of power. When I did my self-initiation ritual, the yolk turned to radiant gold. The real power was recognizing that I had the authority to initiate myself into a new way of being. The power is inside of us. I just needed to remember, and I felt an immediate shift once my ritual was complete.

As you enter the thresholds to heal and reclaim your power, I hope you are inspired to create your own self-initiation ritual. It can be elaborate or simple. The essential ingredient in creating your initiation ritual is that it has meaning for you. Keep the details of your ceremony close to your heart and only share them with those who you trust can fully and unconditionally support you. As I mentioned before, not everything sacred needs to be shared. Some things are just for you and your soul. You may find, as I have, that life will present many thresholds to be acknowledged and honored in your own unique way.

SELF-INQUIRY

To help you move forward with creating your self-initiation ritual, I offer some questions for you to consider. You may also do this initiation more than once;

you always have the power to pause and create a threshold any time you are called.

- What forgotten part of yourself are you ready to remember? *Note: Remember these for the recollection practice below.
- What places make you feel the most powerful and safe? Where should this ritual take place?
- What symbolizes your wounding? How can you reframe that symbol, object, or image to regain your power?
- What element can you employ to transform this image? Examples: earth, bury; water, release in a body of water; fire, burn; air, float, movement; space, explore the void.
- Consider creating an initiation statement or affirmation. What words can you speak to reclaim your power? How can you include your Do Word in your initiation statement?
- How can you reclaim your true Self as the wholeness of who you are and leave behind the false self, the parts of your personality that aren't serving your highest good any longer?
- Go back into your journal and make notes of any important insights that you may want to pull forward into this ritual.
- What are you willing to leave behind to be free? *Note: Remember this for the recollection practice below.
- What attributes are you ready to nurture, cultivate, and tend to?
- How can you remember ahimsa (nonharming) toward yourself or others as you create this ritual?
- What attributes are you ready to nurture, cultivate, and tend to? *Note: Remember these for the recollection practice below.
- What is sacred within you that you are ready to recollect?

Take a few moments to write a paragraph detailing how you envision your ritual. Leave nothing out. How does this ritual space interact with your senses? How does it feel, look, smell, or taste? Include your affirmation and any sacred tools, images, or items you need. How much time is required? Write out all the details as best you can. Envisioning the ritual will begin to create momentum. When you feel complete, place the written or sketched-out version of your ritual on your altar until you are ready for your ceremony. Remember, you can add to it at any time. Let yourself meditate and dream about it until you are prepared.

RECOLLECTION OF SELF PRACTICE

(self-paced or 35 minutes)

The Preparation

Let this practice inspire you to remember your wholeness. First, devote some time to reviewing the answers to the questions that are starred above. Look through your journal for the inspirations and important revelations that may have been sparked from previous practices and inquiries. Make notes about what seems important for your journey going forward. What are you leaving behind and what are you reclaiming? One of the most beautiful practices of remembrance is the practice of deep relaxation. The practice of rotating consciousness throughout the body is a preliminary practice of yoga nidra (the yoga of conscious sleep). It can be traced back to the teachings of the Mahanirvana Tantra from the seventeenth century. Some of these practices were known as *nyasa*, which referred to placing, planting, or anointing the body with sacred symbols, mantras, or deities to invoke the remembrance of the body as a sacred temple of divinity.[1] By rotating our consciousness with awareness, we can recollect our inner divinity and light, honoring a deep desire to once again remember our wholeness and true Self. Every practice can be a ritual if we infuse it with devotion and love. Each "planting" or "placing" in a nyasa practice is a ritual. In the act of rotating consciousness—if you bring awareness to sixty-one places in your body and place a mantra, image, or blessing in each place—you have done sixty-one rituals. This practice of deep relaxation is a ritual of reclaiming your true Self.

As we move through the following, you will be asked to "plant" or "place" your own offerings as part of the practice. Before you begin, dedicate a few minutes to reading through the practice.

The Practice

Begin by cleansing your space in a way that is meaningful to you. Consider herbs and plants that have cultural or spiritual significance to you—sacred smokes, incenses, essential oils, or spray—to purify your space.

Create a rest nest to lie in or set a supportive meditative seat for yourself.

Begin by settling into your breath by placing one hand on your heart and your other hand on your belly. As you place your hands on your body, take a moment to honor your body for its magnificence and offer your gratitude. Feel your navel naturally rising and falling with each breath, allowing your chest to become more and more still. Continue watching your navel rise and fall for five more breaths.

Draw three circles of protective light around your body. On the outside of the circles is everything that is falling away. Recall what you are releasing and letting go of, the lessons you are tired of learning, the old patterns, fears, and habits that keep you small.

Now feel into the space inside of the innermost circle.

The inner circle is full of limitless potential. You are resting in this limitless potential; feel or sense yourself inside of the circles, in the space between, in the threshold between releasing what is limiting and recollecting your truth.

All worries and concerns are outside of the three circles. Nothing outside of the circles can penetrate the inner space inside of the limitless potential that you are resting in.

Begin to feel and sense the space inside of your body as empty. Sense that the space inside of your body is inky black, like a dark night sky. From the tips of your toes to the top of your head, from your shoulders all the way to your fingertips, the inside of your body is dark space.

Holding the sense of the dark night sky inside of your body, begin to become aware of the space outside of your body. Feel the space outside of your body about twelve inches away, still inside of the circles of protection. Feel and sense this space as dark night sky, a void space.

Begin to feel the space outside of your body as a void space, and the space inside of your body as a void space. These two spaces of darkness are only separated by a thin layer of your skin. Move awareness from inside of your body to outside of your body, feeling only your skin as the separation between these two spaces of the void. (10 breaths)

Continue being aware of your breath and of the thin layer of skin between the two void spaces. Begin to count your breaths down from fifty-four toward zero. Each time you count down a number, you feel the layer of skin between the inner space and the outer space become thinner and thinner. Each breath dissolves a layer of skin. When you arrive at zero, the skin is completely dissolved. If you lose track of your account, please start back again at fifty-four. (2 minutes)

Experience yourself as luminous darkness, everywhere and anywhere. (2 minutes)

In this luminous darkness you will begin to reassemble your body piece by piece, part by part. As you reassemble, you will also bring the frequency of what you are being rebirthed as. You will slowly begin to reassemble your body anew, reclaiming your power, truth, and beauty. Each time a body part is named, feel and remember all of that which you are reclaiming. Place or plant your remembrance in the body part. You may sense this as words, images, frequency of light, or a sense of knowing and trust. Bring forward this remembrance and infuse it in that body part. With awareness of each body part, feel the anointment of your divine Self. Each body part receives an anointment of the energy of what you are recollecting. If you aren't sure yet what you are recollecting, use your Do Word or love, freedom, inspiration, and divinity. You can also mentally repeat the affirmation *I remember and reclaim my true Self.*

As you mentally awaken awareness at each body part, silently repeat to yourself, *I remember and reclaim my true Self*, imagining that you are reassembling yourself as a goddess or as a temple of divinity.

Move through the parts of your body one by one. Right-hand thumb, index finger, middle finger, ring finger, little finger, wrist, forearm, elbow, upper arm, shoulder. Left-hand thumb, index finger, middle finger, ring finger, little finger, wrist, forearm, elbow, upper arm, shoulder, throat center, tip of your tongue, openings of your nostrils, bridge of your nose, eyes, third-eye point, forehead, crown of your head, nape of your neck, shoulder blades, spine, sacrum, buttocks, hips, upper legs, knees, lower legs, ankles, soles of your feet. Left your big toe, second toe, third toe, fourth toe, fifth toe, then your right big toe, second toe, third toe, fourth toe, fifth toe. Both feet, both legs, hips, abdomen, navel center, solar plexus, chest, heart center, neck and throat, jaw, lips, cheeks, ears and temples, eyes and eyebrows, third-eye point, crown of your head, whole body, whole body, whole body.

Observe your whole body breathing. (2 minutes)

Allow your awareness to rest at the center of your heart, the abode of your luminous Self at the spiritual heart, deep beneath the breast bone. Let go of all doing and rest in spacious awareness. (3–10 minutes)

Observe the space between resting and waking. Observe your whole body breathing, from the top of your head to the tip of your toes. Remember yourself as a vessel of divinity and grace.

Place your hand on your heart and repeat the mantra SO HAM—"I am that"—or any sacred affirmation that has meaning to you.

Feel and sense this new vibration, the result of the vision, to recreate from your higher consciousness. The courage to dissolve yourself and reassemble yourself in any given moment—that is your power.

When you feel ready, be aware of the space your body occupies and the space around your body. Slowly begin to deepen your breath. Devote a few moments to offer gratitude and the fruits of your practice toward the healing of the collective. Then devote five to ten minutes to freewriting, journaling, or drawing.

Suggested Sadhana

Practice this daily, along with journaling or freewriting, for forty days. After listening to the recording a few times, you may begin to know the general steps of the practice by heart. I encourage you to self-guide yourself through this practice anytime you feel the desire to remember your true Self.

Thank you for spending this time in exploration of your truth, power, and beauty. I hope you have found remembrance, and healing in these pages.

> May we remember who we truly are
> May that memory be a healing
> May we trust our hearts calling
> May we rest in our true nature
> May we love each other
> May we be free

Acknowledgments

My deepest gratitude and love:

To my beloved Harley, who is my biggest supporter and greatest love. Thank you for protecting and honoring my creative cave.

To all teachers who have graciously shared their wisdom and love, especially Swami Veda Bharati, Pandit Rajmani Tigunait, Gary Kraftsow, Swami Prema Jyoti, Laura Amazzone, Uma Dinsmore-Tuli, Elder Malidoma Somé, and Rod Stryker.

To my family, whose love is a healing salve, especially my mother, Dr. Janice Freeman, Harold, Fred, Monique, Sam, Andrew, Katie, Brenda, Baron, and Dane.

To the ancestors: Frederick S. Stanley II, Rev. Louise Ellison, Elder Carl B. Clark, and Kat Alexander.

To Maggie Eileen for the beautiful sacred illustrations.

To loving friends who inspire with laughter and wisdom—the entire ELC community, Deborah Anderson, Chanti Tacoronte-Perez, Mary Bruce, Octavia Raheem, Michelle Cassandra Johnson, Kim Krans, Elena Brower, and Ajit Joshi.

To Alison Beckner, Shannon Ryan, and Cheyann Benedict for the sacred space to create.

To Sari Gelzer, Crystal Marie Higgins, and Deanna Michalopoulous for your support and love.

To Jessica Levine for your sharp eye and warm heart.

And to the team at Shambhala—thank you to my editor Beth Frankl, copyeditor Emily Wichland, and assistant editor Samantha Ripley, as well as designer Kate White, who did the stunning cover art and interior design.

Additional Practices

PRANAYAMA PRACTICES

Ujjayi (Victorious) Breathing

Sealing your lips, allow your jaw to be relaxed. Begin to breathe in and out from your nostrils, feeling a smooth and even stream of breath in and out. Begin to slightly constrict the back of your throat (as though you are trying to fog a mirror with your breath) and notice the sound of your breath become more resonant. This pranayama can be done in any position anytime.

Breath Ratios

These are ways of measuring and portioning the length of your breath, just as you would in a cooking recipe. For example, 1:1 would mean an equal count on both inhale and exhale, whereas 1:2 would mean the exhale is twice the length of the inhale. The inhale represents the number on the left, and exhale is the number on the right. One-to-one breathing is known as *sama vritti* (equal fluctuations), which helps to calm the mind. One-to-two breathing helps to self-regulate by activating the parasympathetic nervous system.

MOVEMENT PRACTICES

Gentle Yoga Asana (10 minutes)

Begin in Makarasana (Crocodile Pose) with 1:2 ratio breathing (ex., inhale 4, exhale 8)

Lying twists
Balasana (Child's Pose) (5 breaths)
Hip circles on all fours (in both directions)
Standing hip circles (in both directions)
Utkata Konasana (Goddess Pose)
Malasana (Garland Pose)
Dynamic Apanasana (Knees to Chest)
Dynamic Dwi Pada Pitham (Bridge Pose)
Lying twist
Savasana (Corpse Pose)

Agnisara Kriya

Agnisara kriya is one of the six cleansing techniques mentioned in the *Hatha Yoga Pradipika*. *Agni* means "sacred fire," and *sara* means "essence." This kriya is wonderful for digestion, assimilation, and processing of physical, emotional, and spiritual matter.

The practice can be done from a standing position or while seated in a chair if you prefer. With knees bent, rest your hands on your knees and lean forward slightly, allowing your pelvis to come into a slight anterior pelvic tilt as you inhale. Your abdominal muscles are pulled in and up on exhalation as you also engage *mula bandha* (root lock). Holding your breath out, deepen the pull of your abdominal wall in and up. When you are ready to release, soften your belly first, then inhale.

Soul Whisper Meditation

Before you settle in for your practice, make sure you have the materials you need to transcribe the wisdom you receive: a notepad, voice recorder, sketch pad, or journal. Give yourself permission to write, draw, or record at any point in the practice. After you are done with the practice, spend a few moments tuning in, getting still, and closing your eyes or doing whatever helps to go inward. Let your awareness rest at the heart center; feel what is there; and hear, feel, see, or sense a deeper part of yourself. Spend two minutes freewriting, drawing, or recording. Don't edit or worry about if it makes logical sense to you at the moment. Just let it flow. Now without looking at your notes, ask yourself, *What is my soul whispering to me?* Then translate (words, image, colors—whatever captures the essence of the message) that in the whisper of the soul circle.

Mental Alarm Clock Practice

Since I learned this practice more than twenty year ago, I have rarely used an alarm clock. Try it:

Before going to sleep, note the time. Close your eyes and visualize the time as it would appear on an analog clock face. See the hands of the clock begin to move until they arrive at the time when you would like to get up. Pause as you see the hands of the clock at that time and repeat silently to yourself, *I will wake up at ___ o'clock.* Then go to sleep. The key to this practice is to let go. It's not a competition or something to get perfect. Go into this practice with a sense of curiosity so you are not up all night checking the clock!

Glossary

abhinivesha Fear of death, clinging to life, and self-preservation. See page 37.

abyhasa Devoted practice with the aim of the final goal of yoga. See page 41.

ahimsa Nonviolence toward others; one of the five yamas described in Patan-jali's Yoga Sutras. See page 74.

annamaya kosha The physical and first layer of energy that covers the soul.

aparigraha Nongreed; one of the five yamas described in Patanjali's Yoga Sutras. See page 75.

asmita Outer sense of "I-am-ness," or egoism, which keeps us distracted, caus-ing us to neglect tending to the inner Self; considered one of the five kleshas, or afflictions, that cause us pain. See page 36.

asteya Nonstealing; one of the five yamas described in Patanjali's Yoga Sutras. See pages 74–75.

avidya Misperception, ignorance, wrong knowledge; considered the cause of suffering, according to Patanjali's Yoga Sutras. See page 33.

bandhas Locks; referring to energy locks done with the physical body to help redirect the flow of prana to specific places in the body. See pages 89–91.

bhakti yoga Yoga of devotion. See page 133.

bija mantra A single-syllable sound that affects a chakra or the subtle body. See page 27.

bodhichitta Completely open heart and mind; *bodhi* means "awake"; *chitta* means "heart/mind." See page 71.

brahmacharya Moderation of the senses and right use of energy; one of the five yamas described in Patanjali's Yoga Sutras. See page 75.

buddhi Discernment; higher or divine intelligence; to wake or be awake. See page 72.

chakras Energy centers of the subtle body. See page 56.

chidakasha Space of pure consciousness or inner space that is beyond thought. See page 113.

core frequency The vibration of one's true Self or eternal essence. See page 53.

devalaya The space the body occupies.

dharana One-pointed focus; the sixth of yoga's eight limbs. See page 110.

dhyana Meditation where the mind is focused on its resting place or origin; the seventh of yoga's eight limbs. See page 110.

dominant culture A culture that has established its own values, hierarchy, and preferences that are imposed as a standard among other people with varying cultures and beliefs. See page xii.

dvesha Sanskrit for aversion, hate, or repulsion toward what we consider to be undesirable. See page 35.

freewriting The act of processing experiences through writing—quickly without concern for sentence structure, grammar, or spelling; deepens understanding and cultivates memory and retentive power (*smriti*). See page 10.

granthi Doubt, shackle, knot. Psychic knots that reside in the subtle body that are obstacles to spiritual enlightenment. See page 85.

hiranyagarbha The cosmic egg, or the golden or universal womb; the golden place inside each of us, a seed of light that contains the entire universe. See page 146.

householder A spiritual practitioner living in the world as opposed to an ashram or hermitage; their primary concerns relates to the upkeep of their home, family, or career while having a spiritual sadhana. See page xv.

hridaya guha The cave of the heart, where a microcosm of the entire universe exists. See page 87.

jnana yoga the yoga of knowledge. See page 108.

karma yoga Yoga of selfless service. See page 43.

kleshas Poisons; used in yogic teachings to describe the five "seeds of affliction" that cause us pain. See page 32.

krama Wise progression or succession. See page 82.

kriya Action or practice combining visualization, mantra, and pranayama; practice that directly affects subtle energy. See page 162.

laya yoga The yoga of dissolution that leads to union with the Divine or *samadhi*, the final goal of yoga. See page 24.

namarupa The self beyond name and form, what makes up our living being. *Nama* is the mental aspect, and *rupa* is the physical form. See page x.

niyamas Five ethical principles in yogic teachings that govern our relationship with ourselves. See page 73.

nonviolent communication Learning to hear our own deeper needs and those of others as a way to discover the depth of compassion. See page 45.

nyasa Placing, planting, or anointing the body with sacred symbols, mantras, or deities. A practice rooted in the consecration of the body as a sacred vessel. See page 154.

panchamahabhutas The five great elements that form the basis of all creation—earth, water, fire, wind, space/ether. See page 54.

Patanjali A sage, said to have been born sometime between the second and fourth centuries C.E., who codified the oral teachings of the ancient rishis into the Yoga Sutras. See page 16.

post-lineage yoga A term coined by Theodora Wildcroft, PhD; a reevaluation of the authority to determine practice and a privileging of peer networks over pedagogical hierarchies or sanghas (communities) over guru-disciple relationships.

pranayama Practices that lead to the expansion of the animating or vital life force; *prana* meaning "animating force," and *ayama* meaning "expansion." See page 161.

praptipaksha bahvana Cultivating the opposite. Yoga Sutra 2:33. See page 39.

pratyahara Withdrawal of the senses so that we can reassimilate into our true nature; the fifth of yoga's limbs. See page 110.

raga Attachment to what is desirable. See page 34.

rishis/rishika The original seers or sages of yoga. See page 16.

sadhana Spiritual practice done consistently over a long time with devotion—for example, daily for forty to ninety days. See page 80.

samadhi Union with the Divine; universal and individual consciousness unite; the final goal of yoga and the eightth of yoga's eight limbs. See page 66.

samskara Impression or imprint made by life experiences that contributes to the makeup of our mental and emotional conditioning; *sam* means "joined together," and *kara* means "action, cause." See page 17.

sangha Like-minded community. See page 74.

satya Truthfulness; one of the five yamas described in Patanjali's Yoga Sutras. See page 74.

Self-devotion Dedicating time and energy to practices to free yourself from pain and suffering in order to touch the wisdom of the true Self. See page 95.

self-initiation The rite of passage experienced when one has a transformative experience brought about by intentional practices of healing. See page 00.

self-inquiry A process of bringing attention to one's innermost thoughts and inner awareness. See page 152.

shruti Sanskrit for "that which is heard via divine revelation." The shruti is also a musical instrument that provides a drone with series of sounds and vibrations produced by bellows.

smarana Constant remembrance of the Divine. See page 82.

smriti Memory or retention; one of the five methods to reach samadhi according to the Yoga Sutras. See page 53.

sutra Thread or suture; with the same Latin root as the English word *suture*, sutra is specifically used to describe the threads woven through the text of Patanjali's Yoga Sutras that connect and build on wisdom that reveals truth. See page 16.

svapna Dream state. See page 131.

tapas The transformative heat produced by the friction of going against the grain of habit and conditioning The heat ignites an inner glow. See page 142.

tapasya A practice that generates the heat of transformation. See page 102.

tattvas The five elements—that is, earth, water, fire, air, and ether/space. See page 24.

tonglen Giving and receiving; the Buddhist practice of compassion and loving-kindness. See page 70.

vairagya Dispassion, detachment, or transparency. See page 40.

vasana Accumulation of imprints that form a coloring in the mind that eventually creates habits. See page 18.

vayu Wind or an energetic force in the body. See page 54.

vichara The practice of deliberation, reflection, and contemplation of ultimate truth that leads to the realization of the true Self. See page 43.

viveka Discriminative wisdom. See page 41.

viyoga The act of separating or subtracting the mind from the senses and sensory objects. See page 66.

witness consciousness A level of awareness characterized by detached, neutral observation of one's own thoughts and feelings. See page 12.

yamas Five ethical principles in yogic teachings that inspire and inform how we treat others. The Sanskrit word *yama* comes from the root word *yam*, which means "to hold back" or "to turn away." See page 73.

yoga To yoke; from the Sanskrit root word *yuj*, meaning "union." See page x.

yoga nidra The practice of conscious sleep where the thread of conscious awareness weaves through all of the states of consciousness; from that rested place, prana guides us back to our source. See page 125.

Notes

INTRODUCTION

1. Explore various translations of this sutra and find a translation that resonates.
2. Swami Prabhavananda and Christopher Isherwood, *How to Know God: The Yoga Aphorisms of Patanjali* (Hollywood, CA: Vedanta Press, 1953), 71.
3. Mukunda Stiles, *Yoga Sutras of Patanjali* (Newburyport, MA: Red Wheel/Weiser, 2021), 12.
4. Ramana Maharshi, *How to Practice Self Inquiry* (N.p.: Freedom Religion Press, 2014).
5. Sobonfu Somé, "Embracing Grief," accessed January 20, 2023, www.sobonfu.com/articles/writings-by-sobonfu2/embracing-grief.
6. Prem Prakash, *The Yoga of Spiritual Devotion: A Modern Translation of the Narada Bhakti Sutras* (Rochester, VT: Inner Traditions International, 1998), 134.
7. Jason Birch and Jacqueline Hargreaves, "Yoganidrā," The Luminescent, January 6, 2015, www.theluminescent.org/2015/01/yoganidra.html.

CHAPTER 1: THAT WHICH MAKES YOU FALL IS THAT WHICH MAKES YOU RISE

1. Swami Veda Bharati, *Yoga Sutras of Patanjali with the Exposition of Vyasa*, Vol. 1, *Samadhi-Pada* (Honesdale, PA: Himalayan International Institute of Yoga Science and Philosophy, 1986), 140.

2. Not everyone is visual. When I invite you to "imagine," you may also feel, sense, or trust.

3. David Berceli, "Neurogenic Tremors," TRE, accessed January 20, 2023, www.omnibalance.se/en/tre%C2%AE/neurogenic-tremors-11655567.

4. Inge Sengelmann, "Shake, Sweat, Tremble and Cry: It's a Bleeping Global Pandemic!" Therapy Aid Coalition, accessed January 20, 2023, https://therapyaid.org/blog/shake-sweat-tremble-and-cry-it-s-a-bleeping-global-pandemic.

5. Jalal al-Din Rumi, "Childhood Friends," in *The Essential Rumi*, trans. Coleman Barks, with John Moyne, A. J. Arberry, and Reynold Nicholson (San Francisco: HarperSanFrancisco, 1995), 142.

CHAPTER 2: YOU ARE NOT YOUR PERSONALITY

1. Kendra Cherry, "What Is Personality?" VeryWellMind, last modified November 7, 2022, www.verywellmind.com/what-is-personality-2795416.

2. Read your favorite translation of Yoga Sutra 1:36, *viśokā vā jyotiṣmatī*.

3. Megan Dalia-Camina, "The Reality of Imposter Syndrome," Psychology Today, September 3, 2018, www.psychologytoday.com/us/blog/real-women/201809/the-reality-imposter-syndrome#:~:text=The%20imposter%20syndrome%20is%20a,being%20exposed%20as%20a%20fraud.

4. Ethan Siegel, "Astrophysics Reveals the Origins of the Human Body," *Forbes*, December 18, 2017, www.forbes.com/sites/startswithabang/2017/12/18/astrophysics-reveals-the-origin-of-the-human-body/?sh=49b591c830a5.

CHAPTER 3: BURNING THE SEEDS OF SORROW— THE POWER OF OPPOSITES

1. Listen to "Self-Care Rituals with Indu Arora," *Radiant Rest*, episode 7, 45:15, www.radiantrest.com/episode-7-self-care-rituals-with-indu-arora/ for more.

2. Swami Veda Bharati, *Yoga Sutras of Patanjali, with the Exposition of Vyasa*, vol. 2 (New Delhi: Motilal Banarsidass, 2009), 74.

3. Nischala Devi, *The Secret Power of Yoga: A Woman's Guide to the Heart and Spirit of the Yoga Sutras*, (New York: Three Rivers Press, 2007), 117.

4. Swami Veda Bharati, *Yoga Sutras of Patanjali, with the Exposition of Vyasa*, vol. 1, *Samadhi-Pada* (Honesdale, PA: Himalayan Institute of Yoga Science and Philosophy, 1986), 102.

5. Reverend Jaganath Carrera, "Patanjali's Words: Pratipaksha Bhavana," accessed January 20, 2023, https://integralyogamagazine.org/patanjalis -words-pratipaksha-bhavana.

6. This line of inquiry is inspired by Carol Iron Rope Herrera, a late Lakota elder.

7. Swami Satyananda Saraswati, *Four Chapters on Freedom* (Munger, India: Yoga Publications Trust, 2013), 91.

8. Bharati, *Yoga Sutras of Patanjali*, 140.

CHAPTER 4: AWAKENING OUR ELEMENTAL NATURE

1. Adrian Alexander, *How Does Historic Trauma Impact Blacks Swimmers?* PACEsConnection, June 21, 2021, https://www.pacesconnection.com/g/ Caribbean/blog/how-does-historic-trauma-impact-blacks-swimmers.

2. The five elements are known as the five tattvas. The whole universe is governed and subsists of earth, air, fire, water, space/ether. On a deeper level, this forms part of the basis of Samkhya's philosophy.

3. Harish Johari, *Chakras* (Rochester, VT: Destiny Books, 2000), 71.

CHAPTER 5: RECOLLECTION AND RECONCILIATION

1. The first iPhone was released in 2007.

2. J. I. Baker, "Digital-Era Brain," *Time Special Edition: The Science of Memory* (New York: Life Books, 2018).

3. Swami Veda Bharati, *Smirti Yoga: Yoga for Memory* (Rishikesh, India: Himalayan Yoga Publications Trust, 2007), 11.

4. John O'Donohue, *To Bless the Space between Us: A Book of Blessings* (New York: Doubleday, 2008), 104.

5. Zahabiyah Yamasaki, email correspondence with the author, August 30, 2022.

CHAPTER 6: THE DO LIST

1. "Granthi," Yogapedia, last modified July 26, 2017, www.yogapedia.com/definition/5291/granthi.

2. David Frawley, "Hridaya Granthi: Releasing the Knots of the Heart," American Institute of Vedic Studies, March 17, 2022, www.vedanet.com/releasing-the-knots-of-the-heart-hridaya-granthi.

3. Swami Swahananda, *Chandogya Upanishad, and Brihadaranyaka Upanishad with Short Commentaries* (CreateSpace Independent Publishing Platform, 2016), 12.

4. David Frawley, "The Mantric Approach of the Vedas," American Institute of Vedic Studies, February 24, 2017, www.vedanet.com/the-mantric-approach-of-the-vedas.

5. David Frawley, "Releasing the Knots of the Heart: Hridaya Granthi," American Institute of Vedic Studies, March 17, 2022, www.vedanet.com/releasing-the-knots-of-the-heart-hridaya-granthi/2022.

6. Swami Muktibodhananda, *Hatha Yoga Pradipika* (Munger, India: Yoga Publications Trust, 1985), 271.

7. Muktibodhananda, *Hatha Yoga Pradipika*, 258.

CHAPTER 7: THE AUSPICIOUS MIND MAP

1. This mind map is inspired and modified from teachings of Isabelle Du Soliel, PhD; personal notes from Yoga of Fulfillment training with Rod Stryker.
2. Cornelia H. M. van Jaarsveld, Henry W. W. Potts, and Jane Wardle, "How Are Habits Formed: Modelling Habit Formation in the Real World," *European Journal of Social Psychology* 40, no. 6 (July 2009): 998–1009.
3. Malidoma Patrice Somé, *Healing Wisdom of Africa: Finding Life Purpose through Nature, Ritual, and Community* (New York: Jeremy P. Tarcher / Putnam, 1998), 160.

CHAPTER 8: EMBRACING TRANSITION

1. Author's personal notes from American Viniyoga Institute Heart-Mind Retreat, led by Gary Kraftsow, Austin, TX, December 2019.
2. Malidoma Patrice Somé, *Ritual: Power, Healing and Community* (New York: Arkana, 1993), 78.
3. Swami Veda Bharati, *Yoga Sutras of Patanjali, with the Exposition of Vyasa,* vol. 1, *Samadhi-Pada* (Honesdale, PA: Himalayan Institute of Yoga Science and Philosophy, 1986), 140.
4. Chandrasekharendra Saraswati, *Hindu Dharma: The Universal Way of Life* (Mumbai, India: Bharatiya Vidya Bhavan, 1995).
5. Anonymous, *The One Lamp That Lights the Worlds: A Translation of the Avadhuta Gita of Dattatreya* (self-pub., 2021).
6. Definition of *pratyahara* from Swami Veda Bharati from personal notes.
7. Read various translations of Vijnana Bhairava Tantra, dharana 52.

CHAPTER 9: THE ANCESTORS HAVE YOUR BACK

1. Joan Halifax, *The Fruitful Darkness* (New York: Grove Press, 1993), 190.

2. Kr. Fateh Singh Jasol, *The Bhagavad Gita: A New Verse Translation* (Chennai, India: Notion Press, 2021), 64.

3. See Dora L. Costa, Noelle Yetter, and Heather DeSomer, "Intergenerational Transmission of Paternal Trauma among US Civil War Ex-POWs," *PNAS* 115, no. 44 (October 15, 2018): 11215–20, www.pnas.org/doi/10.1073/pnas.1803630115.

4. Warren Hooley, "Deepening Our Relationship with the Land," May 26, 2022, https://traceeyoga.com/upcoming-events-yoga/2022/5/26/deepening-our-relationship-with-the-land-practice-and-conversation-with-tracee-stanley-and-warren-hooley.

5. Listen to the audiobook edition of *Of Water and the Spirit: Ritual, Magic, and Initiation of an African Shaman* by Malidome Patrice Somé, read by the author (Novato, CA: New World Library, 2013), 3 hrs.

6. Halifax, *The Fruitful Darkness*, 191.

7. Malidoma Patrice Somé, *Of Water and the Spirit* (New York: Penguin Books, 1994). Audiobook.

8. Yoli Maya Yeh, email correspondence with the author, August 7, 2022.

9. This practice is loosely based on the Vedic practice of *tarpana*. The full practice of tarpana is a nuanced practice that uses specific mantras and mudras and should be guided by your teacher. See https://drsvoboda.com/courses/tantra-courses/ancestors-tarpana-and-shraddha.

CHAPTER 10: DREAM WISDOM

1 Swami Sivanada Radha, *Realities of the Dreaming Mind: The Practice of Dream Yoga* (Spokane, WA: Timeless Books, 2004), 4.

2. Salvador Dali's *The Persistence of Memory*, Mary Shelley's *Frankenstein*, and Larry Page's Google were inspired by dreams.

3. Embodied Philosophy, "What Is Svapna?" December 4, 2019, www.youtube.com/watch?v=c6hIWgGB-90.

4. Sri Aurobindo, *Letters on Yoga: Part Four*, vol. 24 (Pondicherry, India: All India Press, 1970), 1481.

5. A. S. Dalal, comp., *Yoga of Sleep and Dreams/The Night School of Sadhana: Selections from the Works of Sri Aurobindo and the Mother* (Twin Lakes, WI: Lotus Press, 2004), xxiii.

6. Rebecca Renner, "The Pandemic Is Giving People Vivid, Unusual Dreams. Here's Why," *National Geographic*, April 15, 2020, www.national geographic.com/science/article/coronavirus-pandemic-is-giving-people -vivid-unusual-dreams-here-is-why; Brook Jarvis, "Did Covid Change How We Dream?" *New York Times Magazine*, November 4, 2021, www .nytimes.com/2021/11/03/magazine/pandemic-dreams.html; Colleen Walsh, "When You Dream of Feeling Naked in Public—without a Mask," *Harvard Gazette*, May 7, 2021, https://news.harvard.edu/gazette /story/2021/05/how-our-dreams-have-adjusted-to-the-pandemic/.

7. Read Yoga Sutra 3:37.

8. Andrew Holecek, *Dream Yoga: Illuminating Your Life through Lucid Dreaming and the Tibetan Yogas of Sleep* (Boulder, CO: Sounds True, 2016), 37.

9. This is known as the hypnopompic state (Hypnos, the Greek god of sleep; *pompe*, "sending away from"), a transitional state between waking and sleeping.

10. Personal email correspondence with Chanti Tacoronte-Perez, email correspondence with the author, September 5, 2022.

CHAPTER 11: YOU ARE LUMINOUS, WE ARE LUMINOUS

1. David Frawley, "The Ancient Yoga of the Sun," Trust Yoga, accessed January 20, 2023, www.trustyoga.com.sg/knowledge_hub/the-ancient-yoga -of-the-sun-by-david-frawley.

2. Read your favorite translation of Yoga Sutra 1:36.

3. David Frawley, "The Original Teachings of Yoga: From Patanjali Back to Hiranyagarbha," American Institute of Vedic Studies, February 1, 2019, www.vedanet.com/the-original-teachings-of-yoga-from-patanjali-back-to-hiranyagarbha/2019.

4. Michael Meade, "Earth Day Cosmology," *Living Myth*, episode 276, www.mosaicvoices.org/episode-276-earth-day-cosmology.

CHAPTER CONCLUSION: INITIATE YOURSELF— RITUALS OF POWER

1. Arthur Avalon, *Maha Nirvana Tantra: Tantra of Great Liberation* (Create Space Independent Publishing Platform, 2008), 56.

Bibliography

Aggarwal, K. K., and Padma Shri Awardee. "The Main Principle of Knowing the Truth—Neti Neti (Not This, Not This)." *HealthySoch*. August 25, 2019, www.healthysoch.com/health/general/the-main-principle-of-knowing -the-truth-neti-neti-not-this-not-this.

Anderson, Deborah, dir. *Women of the White Buffalo.* Los Angeles: West-mount Pictures, 2022.

Anderson, Sandra. "Guide to Agni Sara." Yoga International. Accessed April 17, 2023. https://yogainternational.com/article/view/guide-to-agni-sara.

Anonymous. *The One Lamp That Lights the Worlds: A Translation of the Avadhuta Gita of Dattatreya.* Self-published, 2021.

Arya, Pandit Usharbudh. *Mantra and Meditation.* Honesdale, PA: Hima-layan Institute Press, 1981.

Aurobindo, Sri, and the Mother. *The Psychic Being: Soul—It's Nature, Mission and Evolution.* Compiled by A. S. Dalal. Wilmot, WI: Lotus Light Press, 1989.

Avalon, Arthur, trans. *Mahanirvana Tantra: Tantra of Great Liberation.* Self-published, CreateSpace, 2008.

———. *The Serpent Power: The Secrets of Tantric and Shaktic Yoga.* New York: Dover Publications, 1974.

Baker, J. I. "Digital-Era Brain." *Time Special Edition: The Science of Memory.* New York: Life Books, 2018.

Berceli, David. "Neurogenic Tremors." TRE. www.omnibalance.se/en/tre%C2%AE/neurogenic-tremors-11655567.

Bharati, Swami Veda. *The Light of Ten Thousand Suns.* Full Circle Publishing, 2009.

———. *Smirti Yoga: Yoga for Memory.* Rishikesh, India: Himalayan Yoga Publications Trust, 2007.

———. *Wanam: Africa and India.* Rishikesh, India: Himalayan Yoga Publications Trust, 2009.

———. *Yoga Sutras of Patanjali, with the Exposition of Vyasa*, Vol. 1, *Samadhi-Pada.* Honesdale, PA: Himalayan Institute Press, 1986.

Birch, Jason, and Jacqueline Hargreaves. "Yoganidra; An Understanding of the History and Context." The Luminescent. January 6, 2015. www.theluminescent.org/2015/01/yoganidra.html.

Bonnasse, Pierre. *Yoga Nidra Meditation: Sleep of the Sages.* Translated by Karina Bharucha. Rochester, VT: Inner Traditions, 2017.

Cherry, Kendra. "What Is Personality?" VeryWellMind. November 7, 2022. www.verywellmind.com/what-is-personality-2795416.

Chödrön, Pema. *When Things Fall Apart: Heart Advice for Difficult Times.* Boulder, CO: Shambhala Publications, 2016.

Coulter, David. "Uddiyana Bandha Step by Step." Yoga International. https://yogainternational.com/article/view/uddiyana-bandha-step-by-step.

Dalal, A. S., comp. *Yoga of Sleep and Dreams/The Night School of Sadhana: Selections from the Works of Sri Aurobindo and the Mother.* Twin Lakes, WI: Lotus Press, 2004.

Dalla-Camina, Megan. "The Reality of Imposter Syndrome." September 3, 2018. www.psychologytoday.com/us/blog/real-women/201809/the-reality-imposter-syndrome#:~:text=The%20imposter%20syndrome%20is%20a,being%20exposed%20as%20a%20ofraud.

Devi, Nischala. *The Secret Power of Yoga: A Woman's Guide to the Heart and Spirit of the Yoga Sutras.* Rev. ed. New York: Harmony Books, 2022.

Divine Life Society. "Bhastrika." Accessed January 20, 2023. https://www .sivanandaonline.org//?cmd=displaysection&section_id=1322.

Frawley, David. "The Mantric Approach of the Vedas." American Institute of Vedic Studies. February 24, 2017. www.vedanet.com/the-mantric -approach-of-the-vedas/.

———. "Our True Self as the Space of Consciousness (Chidakasha)." American Institute of Vedic Studies. March 14, 2022. www.vedanet.com/our -true-self-as-the-space-of-consciousness-chidakasha/2022/.

———. "Releasing the Knots of the Heart: Hridaya Granthi." American Institute of Vedic Studies. March 17, 2022. www.vedanet.com/releasing -the-knots-of-the-heart-hridaya-granthi/.

———. *Vedantic Meditation: Lighting the Flame of Awareness.* Berkeley, CA: North Atlantic Books, 2000.

———. *The Yoga of Consciousness: From Waking, Dream, and Deep Sleep to Self-Realization.* Twin Lakes, WI: Lotus Press, 2020.

Gateway Africa. "Hottentot Deities: Superstitions from Southern Africa." www.gateway-africa.com/stories/Hottentot_Deities.html.

Halifax, Joan. *The Fruitful Darkness: A Journey through Buddhist practice and Tribal Wisdom.* New York: Grove Press, 1993.

Holecek, Andrew. *Dream Yoga: Illuminating Your Life through Lucid Dreaming and the Tibetan Yogas of Sleep.* Boulder, CO: Sounds True, 2016.

Jagadisvaranada, Swami, trans. *Devi Mahatmyam.* Kolkata, India: Advaita Ashram, 2001.

Jarvis, Brooke. "Did Covid Change How We Dream?" *New York Times Magazine,* November 3, 2021. www.nytimes.com/2021/11/03/magazine /pandemic-dreams.html.

Jung, C. G. *The Psychology of Kundalini Yoga: Notes of the Seminar Given in 1932.* Edited by Sonu Shamdasani. Princeton, NJ: Princeton University Press, 1996.

Lakshmanjoo, Swami. *The Manual for Self-Realization: 112 Meditations of the Vijnana Bhairava Tantra*. Damascus, OR: Lakshmanjoo Academy, 2015.

———. *The Mystery of Vibrationless Vibration in Kashmir Shaivism*. Damascus, OR: Lakshmanjoo Academy, 2016.

Le Page, Joseph, and Lilian Le Page. *Mudras for Healing and Transformation*. Sebastopol, CA: Integrative Yoga Therapy, 2014.

Lotzof, Kerry. "Are We Really Made of Stardust?" Natural History Museum. Accessed April 17, 2023. www.nhm.ac.uk/discover/are-we-really-made-of-stardust.html.

Mirabal, Robert, and Nelson Zink. *Believe in the Corn: Manual for Puebloan Corn Growing*. 2011. Kindle.

Mitchell, Stephen, trans. *Bhagavad Gita: A New Translation*. New York: Harmony, 2000.

Momaday, N. Scott. *The Way to Rainy Mountain*. 50th anniv. ed. Albuquerque: University of New Mexico Press, 2019.

Muktibodhanada, Swami. *Hatha Yoga Pradipika*. Munger, India: Yoga Publications Trust, 1985.

Mutwa, Vusamazulu Credo. *Songs of the Stars: The Lore of a Zulu Shaman*. Barrytown, NY: Station Hill Press, 2000.

O'Donohue, John. *To Bless the Space between Us: A Book of Blessings*. New York: Doubleday, 2008.

———. *Four Elements: Reflections on Nature*. New York: Harmony Books, 2010.

Prakash, Prem. *The Yoga of Spiritual Devotion: A Modern Translation of the Narada Bhakti Sutras*. Rochester, VT: Inner Traditions, 1998.

Radha, Swami Sivananda. *Realities of the Dreaming Mind: The Practice of Dream Yoga*. Spokane, WA: Timeless Books, 2004.

Rama, Swami. *Perennial Psychology of the Bhagavad Gita*. Honesdale, PA: Himalayan Institute Press, 1985.

Renner, Rebecca. "The Pandemic Is Giving People Vivid, Unusual Dreams. Here's Why." *National Geographic*, April 15, 2020. www.national

geographic.com/science/article/coronavirus-pandemic-is-giving
-people-vivid-unusual-dreams-here-is-why.

Rosenberg, Stanley. *Accessing the Healing Power of the Vagus Nerve: Self-Help Exercises for Anxiety, Depression, Trauma, and Autism.* Berkeley, CA: North Atlantic Books, 2017.

Rumi, Jalal al-Din. "Childhood Friends." In *The Essential Rumi.* Translated by Coleman Barks. San Francisco: HarperSanFrancisco, 1995.

Sams, Jamie. *Earth Medicine: Ancestor's Ways of Harmony for Many Moons.* San Francisco: HarperSanFrancisco, 1994.

Saraswati, Swami Gyanbhikshu. "Achievement of Yoga in Viyoga." Sanskrit Magazine. Accessed April 17, 2023. www.sanskritimagazine.com/yoga/ achievement-yoga-viyoga/.

Saraswati, Swami Satyasangananda. *Sri Vijnana Bhairava Tantra: The Ascent.* Munger, India: Yoga Publications Trust, 2003.

Sengelmann, Inge. "Shake, Sweat, Tremble and Cry: It's a Bleeping Global Pandemic!" Therapy Aid Coalition. May 11, 2020. https://therapyaid .org/blog/shake-sweat-tremble-and-cry-it-s-a-bleeping-global-pandemic.

Siegel, Ethan. "Astrophysics Reveals the Origin of the Human Body." *Forbes*, December 18, 2017. www.forbes.com/sites/startswithabang/2017/12/18/ astrophysics-reveals-the-origin-of-the-human-body/?sh=6430de3730a5.

Somé, Malidoma Patrice. *Healing Wisdom of Africa: Finding Life Purpose through Nature, Ritual, and Community.* New York: Jeremy P. Tarcher/ Putnam, 1998.

———. *Of Water and the Spirit: Ritual, Magic, and Initation in the Life of an African Shaman.* New York: Penguin, 1994.

———. *Ritual: Power, Healing and Community.* New York: Arkana, 1993.

Sovik, Rolf. "A Beginner's Guide to Mula Bandha." Yoga International. Accessed April 17, 2023. https://yogainternational.com/article/view/a -beginners-guide-to-mula-bandha-root-lock.

Stanley, Tracee. *Radiant Rest: Yoga Nidra for Deep Relaxation and Awakened Clarity.* Boulder, CO: Shambhala Publications, 2021.

Sunderal Dabral, Achraya. "The Science of Mudra" (lecture). Accessed April 17, 2023. https://doczz.net/doc/5207824/the-science-of-mudras.

Tigunait, Pandit Rajmani. *The Practice of the Yoga Sutra: Sadhana Pada.* Honesdale, PA: Himalayan Institute, 2017.

Tigunait, Pandit Rajmani. "The 24 Gurus of Dattatreya." Himalayan Institute. June 8, 2020. https://himalayaninstitute.org/online/the-24-gurus -of-dattatreya/.

Tiwari, Maya. *Women's Power to Heal through Medicine.* Mother Om Media, 2012.

Walsh, Colleen. "When You Dream of Feeling Naked in Public—without a Mask." *Harvard Gazette,* May 7, 2021. https://news.harvard.edu/gazette /story/2021/05/how-our-dreams-have-adjusted-to-the-pandemic/.

Whicher, Ian. *The Integrity of Yoga Darasana: A Reconsideration of Classical Yoga.* New York: State University of New York Press. 1998.

ADDITIONAL LINKS

Embodied Philosophy. "What Is Svapna?" December 4, 2019. www.youtube .com/watch?v=c6hIWgGB-90&ab_channel=EmbodiedPhilosophy.

King, Bernadette. "Air: New Life, Power of the Mind, Communication." Building Beautiful Souls. Accessed April 17, 2023. www.buildingbeautiful souls.com/symbols-meanings/five-elements-symbolic-meaning/air -element-symbolic-meaning/#%20AirSymbolism.

Manorama. "Threading the Sutra." Sanskrit Studies. Accessed April 17, 2023. https://sanskritstudies.org/threading-the-sutra.

Newton, Ivy. "What's Your Dagara Cosmology Sign." African Food History, Art, and Spirituality. Accessed April 17, 2023. www.theafricangourmet .com/2016/07/whats-your-dagara-cosmology-sign.html.

Online Etymology Dictionary, s.v. "reconciliation," last modified May 21, 2021, www.etymonline.com/word/reconciliation.

Recommended Resources

SELF-INQUIRY

Ramana Maharshi. *How to Practice Self Inquiry*. N.p.: Freedom Religion Press. 2014.

AVIDYA

Bharati, Swami Veda. *Yoga Sutras of Patanjali, with the Exposition of Vyasa*. Vol. 2. New Delhi: Motilal Banarsidass, 2001.

Tigunait, Pandit Rajmant. *The Practice of the Yoga Sutra: Sadhana Pada*. Honesdale, PA: Himalayan Institute, 2017.

MIND MAPPING

Stanley, Tracee. "The Ritual of Mind Mapping; Explore How to Bring More Creativity and Inspiration into Your Life." Traceeyoga.com. https://traceeyoga .com/upcoming-events-yoga/2021/10/29/the-ritual-of-mind-mapping.

CHAKRAS AND SUBTLE BODY

Johari, Harish. *Chakras: Energy Centers of Transformation.* Rochester, VT: Destiny Books, 2000.

Little, Tias. *Yoga of the Subtle Body: A Guide to Physical and Energetic Anatomy of Yoga.* Boulder, CO: Shambhala Publications, 2016.

ANCESTORS AND GRIEF

Johnson, Michelle Cassandra. *Finding Refuge: Heartwork for Healing Collective Grief.* Boulder, CO: Shambhala Publications, 2021.

Somé, Malidoma Patrice. *Healing Wisdom of Africa: Finding Life Purpose through Nature, Ritual, and Community.* New York: Jeremy P. Tarcher/Putnam, 1998.

———. *Of Water and the Spirit: Ritual, Magic, and Initation in the Life of an African Shaman.* New York: Penguin, 1994.

DREAMS

Dreaming and Creativity Classes by Chanti Tacoronte-Perez: yantrawisdom.com.

Holecek, Andrew. *Dream Yoga: Illuminating Your Life through Lucid Dreaming and the Tibetan Yogas of Sleep.* Boulder, CO: Sounds True, 2016.

Morley, Charlie. *Dreams of Awakening: Lucid Dreaming and Mindfulness of Dream and Sleep.* London: Hay House, 2013.

Radha, Swami Sivananda. *Realities of the Dreaming Mind: The Practice of Dream Yoga.* Spokane, WA: Timeless Books, 2004

TRAUMA-INFORMED YOGA

Parker, Gail. *Restorative Yoga for Ethnic and Race-Based Stress and Trauma.* London: Singing Dragon, 2020.

Yamasaki, Zahabiyah. *Trauma-Informed Yoga for Survivors of Sexual Assault: Practices for Healing and Teaching with Compassion.* New York: W. W. Norton, 2022.

THERAPISTS

Dr. Hanna Chusid, https://www.drhannachusid.com
Inge Sengelmann, https://embodyyourlife.org
Therapy for Black Girls, https://therapyforblackgirls.com

YOGA NIDRA

Desai, Kamini. *Yoga Nidra: The Art of Transformational Sleep.* Twin Lakes, WI: Lotus Press, 2017.

Dinsmore-Tuli. *Yoga Nidra Made Easy: Deep Relaxation Practices to Improve Sleep, Relieve Stress and Boost Energy and Creativity.* London: Hay House, 2022.

Miller, Richard C. *The iRest Program for Healing PTSD: A Proven-Effective Approach to Using Yoga Nidra Meditation and Deep Relaxation Techniques to Overcome Trauma.* Oakland, CA: New Harbinger Publications, 2015.

Stanley, Tracee. *Radiant Rest: Yoga Nidra for Deep Relaxation and Awakened Clarity.* Boulder, CO: Shambhala Publications, 2021.

About the Author

TRACEE STANLEY is the author of the bestselling book *Radiant Rest: Yoga Nidra for Deep Relaxation and Awakened Clarity* and the founder of Empowered Life Circle, a sacred community and portal of practices, rituals, and Tantric teachings inspired by more than twenty-five years of studentship in Sri Vidya Tantra and the teachings of the Himalayan Masters. As a post-lineage teacher, Tracee is devoted to sharing the wisdom of yoga nidra, rest, meditation, self-inquiry, nature as a teacher, and ancestor reverence. Tracee is gifted in illuminating the magic and power found in liminal space and weaving devotion and practice into daily life. She lives with her husband and two dogs in northern New Mexico. Find out more about Tracee at traceestanley.com.